"...what a delightful and sophisticated content, yet simple to digest. Highly recommendable book, with applicable and practical wellbeing principles. Every parent (present and future) ought to absorb its knowledge."

- Dr. O. Davies

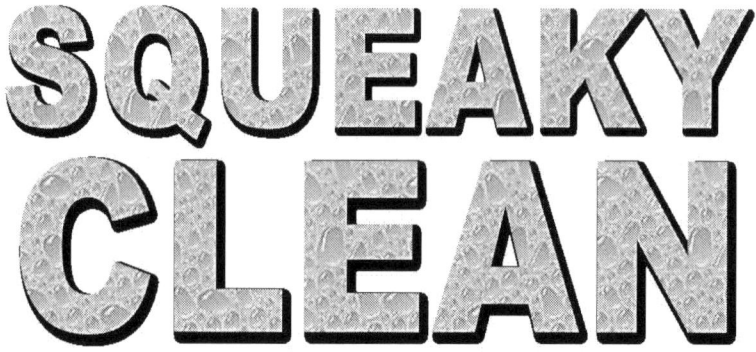

UNIQUE NEWBORN BABY RUBDOWN

By B. JOHNSON OLISENEKU

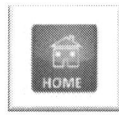

www.squeaky-clean.net

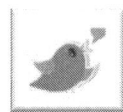

www.twitter.com/squeakyclean_

www.facebook.com/Newbornrubdown

Copyright © 2014 B. Johnson Oliseneku

All rights reserved. No part of this book may be used or reproduced by any means, graphic, electronic, or mechanical, including photocopying, recording, taping or by any information storage retrieval system without the written permission of the publisher except in the case of brief quotations embodied in critical articles and reviews.

Because of the dynamic nature of the Internet, any web addresses or links contained in this book may have changed since publication and may no longer be valid. The views expressed in this work are solely those of the author and do not necessarily reflect the views of the publisher.

The author of this book does not dispense medical advice or prescribe the use of any technique as a form of treatment for physical, emotional, or medical problems without the advice of a physician, directly or indirectly. The intent of the author is only to offer information of a general nature to help you in your quest for emotional and spiritual well-being. In the event you use any of the information in this book for yourself, which is your constitutional right, the author and the publisher assume no responsibility for your actions.

Any people depicted in stock imagery provided by Thinkstock; Dreamtime and Muskat Works are models, and such images are being used for illustrative purposes only.
Certain stock imagery are copyrighted © Thinkstock, Dreamtime and Muskat Works.

Printed in the United States of America

Digital format-distribution available online via Kindle & Nook.

ISBN-13: 978-1500961633 (Coloured interior)
ISBN-13: 978-1500943950 (Monochrome interior)

Rev. Date: 01/07/2015

CONTENTS

DEDICATION IX
FOREWORD XI
PREFACE XIII
INTRODUCTION XIV

CHAPTER ONE………..1
THE NEWBORN BABY 1
Your Baby's First Test 3
Breast-Feeding 4
Taking Your New Baby Home 4

CHAPTER TWO 7
WHAT IS A MASSAGE? 7
Baby Massage, Its Definition? 8
The Origin and History of 'Rubdown' 8
Do Newborn Rubdowns Differ from Infant Massage? . 12

CHAPTER THREE 15
CLINICAL STUDY 15
Research Methodology 16
Research Findings 16

CHAPTER FOUR 19
WHEN TO GIVE A MASSAGE 19
Stress 20
Colic 21

CHAPTER FIVE 25
BENEFITS OF THE UNIQUE NEWBORN RUBDOWN 25

CHAPTER SIX…..….29
HOW TO PERFORM A NEWBORN BABY RUBDOWN..................... 29
Basic Items Required for Newborn Baby Rubdown 31
Demystifying Palm Oil Derivatives 33
Palm Oil in Wound Care 34
Red Palm Oil 34
Refined, Bleached, Deodorized Palm Oil 35
Benefits: Minerals and Vitamin in Lubricants 42
Method Use in Newborn Rubdown 43

v

CHAPTER SEVEN 48
IT'S BATH TIME 48
Getting Ready for Baby's First Bath 48
The Bath 50
Bathtub Time for Baby 54

CHAPTER EIGHT 57
SUBSEQUENT BABY MASSAGE 57
Items Used for the Massage: **Error! Bookmark not defined.**
Newborn Kits 60
An Outdoor Bag with Baby's Essentials 61
Mother and Baby Unit 61

CHAPTER NINE 64
ME TIME 64
Self-Massage 70
Self-Massage Techniques 71

CHAPTER TEN 74
STRESS LINKED TO BIRTH TRAUMA 74
Eliminate Stress 77
Set Realistic Expectations 78
1. The Art of Being Present 85
2. Staying Calm 86
3. Find and Embrace True Clarity 87
4. Find and Use Your Support System 88
5. Effective, Assertive, and Two-Way Communication 89
6. Happier and Stress Free 89
7. Embrace Your Passion 90
8. Time Management 91
9. Reconnect with Sibling at Their Level 92
10. Application of These Concepts 93

SUMMARY 97
General Critique 99

NOTES 101
BIBLIOGRAPHY 102
INDEX 110
ABOUT THE AUTHOR 114

A unique **Newborn Baby massage also called 'Rubdown'** with Special First Bath and many helpful tips for Mothers, specifically, pragmatic approach to better equip mothers against Parenting Stress, with a view to effectively manage time.

DEDICATION

I dedicate this book to my daughter, for her inspirational insight to write a book and, enduring life's challenges with great courage. The statement that life's challenges build endearing characters has a basis on the good and the bad. She is an angel who tackles life's challenges with admiration from those around her. A great support from a strong-minded individual is invaluable with moral implications. It is necessary to take good care of children from birth in order to mould them into honourable individuals, beyond the call of duty. In addition, it takes a 'village' to raise a child, denoting a community of support network of both personal and professional in nature. These essential attributes though, imbued culturally and ethically in our society, and logically perceived as fundamental to being human.

We all have our crosses to bear, but some are more challenging to manage than others. Moreover, the saying of, 'what does not kill one makes one stronger is not far-fetched.' Suffice to mention the rough patches and character building, which led to inspirational encouragement we both shared; this includes being inspired to write this book. The 'overcomer' is a person who has truly experienced what life is about and dealt with both conventional and controversial issues with precision.

A special thank-you goes to all the contributors especially, to the parents and babies who participated and gave their consent, in a brave attempt to advance their knowledge and skills. My special thanks go to a family friend whose mother (deceased after a short illness) introduced me to newborn rubdown. I learned the technique during her visit, and was subsequently able to retain the experience. The procedure has many benefits indeed; it is a concept that even experienced healthcare professionals' battle initially to accept. It is, of course understandable to exercise caution of a newly introduced procedure. The general thought of the idea was submerge subconsciously, until recently, when an 'aha' moment engulfed me. A mixed emotion, at times, can spell doom or success of any idea, even this baby rubdown. In this case, success will emerge at the prospect of sharing this discovery with parents. I can confirm that, having typed out the main structure of this book over a few hours, the rest is history. What a feeling. Finally, a special dedication to newborn babies wherefore, pragmatically, one embraces all cultures and acknowledge a way forward for multi-cultural practises. It is truly possible to advance one's achievement, with faith and strong determination.'

FOREWORD

Newborn babies are treasure to behold and bundle of joy to families, wonderfully created and assurance of prosperity on earth. They are the future! They deserve great and loving care, for their wellbeing, especially good health. Rubdown is one of the ways to achieve these. It is a unique, first and special bath that precedes the first bath for newborn babies and involves the use of oil lubricant, without applying pressure; this makes it different from massage. It is an ancient traditional practice originating in West Africa, a list of impressive benefits for children, nursing mothers and caregivers. However, its continuity is endangered due to lack of knowledge, adoption and global awareness, although, widely known in west of the African continent. Squeaky Clean has a high recommendation for its beneficial appeal, to ensure its worldwide adoption, application and its sustainability. The author is a healthcare professional, with experience that spans over two decades in the private and public healthcare sectors, both in United Kingdom and in Africa.

The present book aptly titled "Squeaky Clean, unique newborn baby massage, known as 'Rubdown' with special first bath and tips for parents, specifically, practical tips to better equip mothers against parenting stress, with a view to effectively manage time." It is unique in its contributions to knowledge in the medical science relating to newborns, infants and nursing mothers. It gives useful and practical tools to improve baby's wellbeing and health. It also provides clinical, cultural and social benefits of the subject matter giving the younger and future generations the opportunity to acquire the knowledge of this ancient procedure. The book has ten chapters with information on baby care and summaries on aspects of birth related stress. The benefits of the "Rubdown" are numerous, clean skin, glowing, radiant, and soft and smooth skin. Other visible benefits are a complete removal of vernix caseosa at birth, relaxed muscles, relief from stress, colic pain, good sleeping regime, promotes growth, development of preterm or low birth-weight infants and aids belching amongst others. Squeaky Clean provides a quick understanding of the content to nursing mothers, caregivers, including, midwives, nurses, paediatricians, medical practitioners and everyone who is inclined to gain relevant knowledge. It is a valuable asset with wealth of relevant information to this generation and the generation yet unborn.

Doctor Onome Davies is a lecturer at the Rivers State University of Science and Technology, Port Harcourt, Nigeria. Retains Post-Doctorate Fellow of African Women in Agricultural Research and Development (AWARD), Fellow of Netherlands Fellowship Programme (NFP).

PREFACE

What a joy for expectant mothers and families to have their desire of a healthy newborn baby. A new addition to a family denotes a new beginning and a great adjustment for mothers, partners, and siblings. Babies deserve a wonderful gift of a lifetime, whether or not one decides to apply the method advocated in "Squeaky Clean". This book primarily teaches the preventative and safe steps to avoid malodorousness and additional tips of subsequent healthy activities. It is a unique, first 'baby rubdown,' incorporating the bath of the newborn baby, which promotes a healthy lifestyle. In addition, learn to apply the secondary procedure to calm baby and release stress, pain, abdominal wind, and many more benefits. It is a known concept that parents can learn this technique before the birth of their babies and can assist others. The implication of failing to heed the advice could lead to an unequivocal impact on the newborn baby beyond childhood.

The primary purpose of this book "Squeaky Clean" is to create awareness of this unique rubdown and the following bathing of newborns, in particular to parents and caregivers. However, it includes a particular focus on the health and well-being of mothers and newborns. In addition, to demonstrate the different methods of massage, together with helpful tips in combating stress particularly, in relation to parenting. My background is in healthcare, spanning three decades, and a women's health expert with a degree in applied social sciences. In my professional life, having acquired numerous postgraduate courses in healthcare, human resources, and leadership; the daily experience of interacting with people from multi-cultural backgrounds is enriching, even in a media setting dubbed 'cultural fusion centre of the world' – that is, London.

INTRODUCTION

This unique book traces the history of the practise of newborn baby rubdown in Africa, as well as, the origin of the proposed oil. The proposal to promote the benefits of the application of this technique from scientific, cultural, and social points of view in order to prevent malodorousness and to explore the ethical promotion of health and well-being. The *Oxford Dictionary* defines malodorousness as 'the state of smelling extremely unpleasant.' Is it a disease, if so; is it treatable? It is not a life-threatening state of consciousness for non-sufferers; but sufferers will beg to differ.

It is a fact that the body's natural smell is non- offensive, and less so with a clean body. However, the combination of bacteria acting on sweat, dirt, and other elements on the body could be provocative and intolerable to the nose. My preventative advocacy within the content of this book is less challenging and better than a cure; ultimately, 'a stitch in time saves nine.'

It is not very often that one has an opportunity to write a book on baby hygiene, and one written in a global context of health and wellbeing. The sheer practicality of acquiring a skill that is both safe for newborns and valuable if applied at the appropriate time is prudish and befitting. Furthermore, this process may ensure that newborns will escape the burden of acquiring preventative body odour beyond childhood. This bath incorporates an application of oil lubricant using a technique similar to massage. The massage and following bath is a handy tool for parents. There is no claim that everyone who did not have this special massage and the subsequent bath after birth has developed malodorousness, and neither does one advocate administering it to all newborn babies. One perceived that the implication of not giving the newborn baby rubdown could result in or aid the process of the likelihood of developing body odour later in adulthood.

In my opinion as a mother and a healthcare professional, by massaging the baby, many parents will be able to help the baby relax, thereby managing many of the common causes of the baby's restlessness. They could display restlessness following birth in view of the new environment, their perception of an alien one (hostile outside the uterus) to their previous development and growth in the uterus. It is standard for babies to cry to alert caregivers if they are hungry, uncomfortable, sick, or in pain. Please note that they will not cry when they are happy, contrary to adults in situations beyond their imagination, such as the birth of a baby or winning the lottery. The latter being the highlights of the tears of joy, often displayed by adults.

I share the joy of being part of many childbirths, parents shedding tears after delivery was considerably standard. It is also normal as a midwife to hold back tears, especially, in view of a teary face misinterpretation. The burden of tackling numerous deliveries could ultimately take its toll, but nonetheless it is a great joy to behold a newborn. At the core of this was the reward of seeing healthy mothers, babies, and families returning home with their bundles of joy. 'Push, push, and push!' I gave all that up, not without the regret of not seeing the births of newborn babies and the joy of parents. The other phrase commonly used in labour by healthcare professionals is, 'Breathe, breathe, breathe.' Of course, they are breathing, but it is a common exercise to occupy women in labour, because it helps to relax them whilst the brain produces endorphins for the pain. Endorphins are natural painkillers produced in the brain. They are endogenous opioid peptides that function as neurotransmitters. They the pituitary gland and the hypothalamus produces it in vertebrates during exercise, excitement, pain, consumption of spicy food, making love and orgasm, and they resemble the opiates in mammals with the ability to produce analgesia and giving a feeling of well-being.

There were wonderful memories whilst practising midwifery, in private and public healthcare sectors, both in the UK and overseas! It is with great endeavour that one explore the opportunities of seemingly greener pasture, which often beckons. The experiences in private and public sectors are similar in various aspects and sometimes overlap in many others. However, having been privileged to experience both, has inspirationally led to writing of this book. It is a personal choice of avenue to share my experience with parents, as a gift and commitment to general healthcare and better lifestyle.

It is a privilege to continue to focus on women's health, and there is no doubt in my mind that other planned projects would succeed regardless of seemingly harmless barriers. Some may call them challenges or merely necessary obstacles', but whatever their purpose and often distractive occurrence, one must persevere in the face of any adversity. This is for all parents, and hopefully, it encourages and inspires you to achieve your goals. The overall purpose of learning by practising those things that are important in life can serve as convenient tools to improve baby's wellbeing. Learning the procedure will enrich one, master it, and pass it on to future generations, or simply share your experience amongst friends and family. It is my sincere hope that parents gain inspiration, by the principles within this book "Squeaky Clean" and truly enjoy its use.

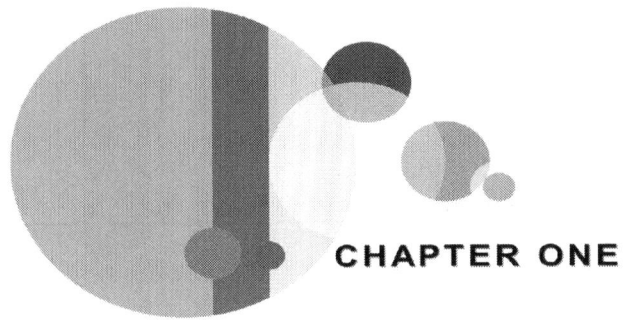

CHAPTER ONE

THE NEWBORN BABY

Congratulations to parents on the birth of their baby, what a bundle to behold! This image of a baby captures a delightful reality experienced by mothers and imagined by others.

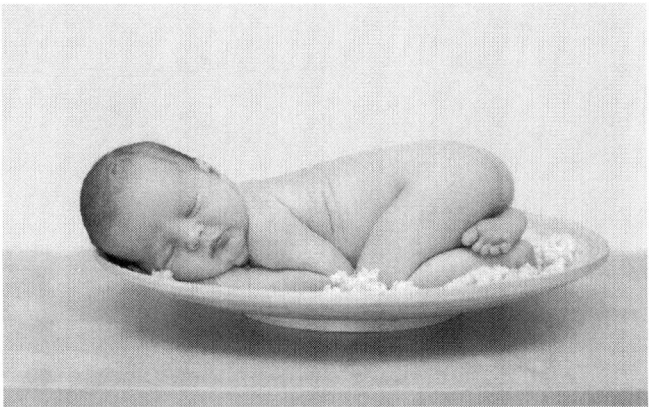

Newborn Baby in a dish

The joy of having a baby is immeasurable for mothers, the experience could probably be the most life-altering yet amazing thing they will ever do. The mother is likely to be elated and exhausted, tired and excited, and a little bit in shock; despite the nine months of preparation, and the baby's first day will undoubtedly bring fond memories. These mixed emotions are priceless, and it is okay to be teary eyed with joy. Nevertheless, what does it feel like to be a new mum, and what should one expect in the first minutes and hours? For a period of approximately nine months, babies are in the confines of the uterus, developing and growing series of tissues, including muscles. Whilst it is a normal process of development in this environment, it is also restrictive for movement. Consequently, at birth the baby undergo a series of checks. This will further ensure that, they have undergone a healthy development following birth.

There are sets of health professionals who may conduct their first checks called the newborn checks. Whilst the paediatrician may carry out the medical checks, the midwife would undoubtedly check the newborn baby; again, this depends on the organisational policy (clinical and non-clinical settings), the mode of delivery, location, culture and society.

> ***Tips***
> *Do not forget to take many snapshots! They are gems in their own rights, capturing unique moments.*

Your Baby's First Test

The APGAR test is carried out when baby is one minute old and again at five minutes to check the appearance, pulse, grimace (her or his response to stimulation), activity, and respiration. The baby will be given a mark out of ten, with a result between seven and ten considered normal. The baby's measurements are recorded, including the circumference of the head and appropriately weighed. All data entered on the developmental chart; is given by the midwife or health visitor as part of the personal child health record to the parent.

Between four and forty-eight hours old, baby will have a full newborn examination. A paediatrician or a midwife will check the heart, hips, and eyes (and for boys, the testicles) as a standard check-up. This is standard in many settings, and thereafter for a five-year period. It is standard in many societies and institutions as part of health and well-being for all children.

The other professionals who may be privileged to check the baby are the general practitioner or medical doctor (GP or MD), or the school nurse. The latter, when they are old enough to attend school. These checks are vital for the baby from birth and onwards, and they need the consent of the mother and the cooperation of the baby for thorough checks or observations that are very essential.

The overall rigour of undergoing childbirth can be very tiring, regardless of the mode of delivery and outcome. It is understandable that parents only want the best for their newborn baby, desiring health and strength in all aspects.

If the mother, being the primary caregiver, has undergone a caesarean section, she may have needed a general anaesthetic and probably; was not conscious during the birth. Some mothers feel very disappointed about this, but organising a birthing review with your carers and talking about your experience and expectations (what happened and why) can help parents come to terms with any issues. I advocate this and urge mothers to take full advantage of the birthing debrief, which can minimise post-natal depression. There is no getting around the fact that a caesarean is major abdominal surgery, and mothers may feel pain afterwards. A stay in the hospital for at least three days is the norm, after an invasive operation mentioned above and working at a minimal pace for six to eight weeks is, clinically normal.

Breast-Feeding

If the mother is well enough and wants to breastfeed the baby, then encouragingly, she can try it within the first hour. There is plenty of support and advice in the hospital to help new mothers get in the right position, and the baby will likely latch on the breast. This is natural for the baby, who can easily navigate to locate his or her food.
  Some babies may need additional assistance to latch on to the breast; however once on, they tend to progress unaided. Did you know it is common fact that mums who suckle their babies shortly after birth have a greater chance of successfully breastfeeding them long-term? Nonetheless, babies are individuals, and patience is crucial when dealing with them. If you struggle with it, learn to be patient – it is an invaluable virtue required for parenting. Breastfeed babies for as long as possible, even beyond toddler age, for a happy and healthy childhood. Babies that are breastfed, scientifically proven, are better able to fight off many childhood illnesses and diseases, due to the immunity in breast milk (WHO 2013).

> *Tips*
> *Mum, be patient and trust your instinct. Some babies may require longer times to latch onto the breast. This is common.*

Taking Your New Baby Home

What could be more natural than taking your baby home? There are several preparations, following discharge, from the hospital; of which parents needs to be aware. First are items that babies will need in their first car ride. If the mode of transport to home is by car, do not forget to use special baby car seat; the law requires it in many societies and countries. The seat should face the rear of the car, and the baby, wrapped up warmly for the journey home, so make sure that a packed blanket is in your hospital bag.

It is a well-known fact that contact between mother and child should not be interrupted during the first hour after birth or until, the mother gives the first breastfeeding, cited by Michel Odent (2002). The importance of maintaining contact between baby and mother at this moment could also facilitate breast-feeding both, in the short and long terms. This view is supported by UNICEF UK (2013), Odent, M. (2002) and research in Sweden, and it is clinically acceptable in the healthcare sector.

> ***Fact***
> *A newborn is an infant who is in the first 28 days after birth.*

CHAPTER TWO

WHAT IS A MASSAGE?

The definition of the term 'massage' in the *Oxford Dictionary* is rubbing and kneading of muscles and joints of the body with the hands or another appliance, mechanical or, otherwise, especially to relieve tension or pain. This definition of course is for the adults, and kneading of muscles and joints does not apply to baby massage. Why does it differ? That is because babies are delicate and fragile, and the methods used by adult would cause injury to babies. The paragraph below describes the definition of baby massage and subsequently the newborn baby rubdown.

Weerapong et al., (MD, sports medicine 2005) further defines massage as the manipulating of superficial and deeper layers of muscle and connective tissue using various techniques. Furthermore, 'to enhance function, aid in the healing process, decrease muscle reflex activity, inhibit motor-neuron excitability, promote relaxation and health, and as a recreational activity' *(Weerapong P. et al., 2005)*. The word comes from the French *massage*, 'friction of kneading,' or from the Arabic *massa*, meaning 'to touch, feel, or handle,' or from the Latin *massa*, meaning 'mass, dough' *(Source Merriam Webster 2014)*. In Oxford dictionary, the word in Greek, *massō*, is 'to handle, touch, to work with the hands, to knead dough.' In distinction, the ancient Greek word for massage was *anatripsis*, and the Latin was *friction*. Massage involves working and acting on the body with pressure-structured, unstructured, stationary, or moving-tension motion or vibration, manually or with mechanical aids. The most cited reasons for introducing massage as therapy in adults have been client demand and perceived clinical effectiveness, cited by Weerapong et al., (2005).

In professional settings, massage involve the client lying on a massage table while being treated, sitting in a massage chair, or lying on a mat on the floor. The massage subject may be fully or partially clothed or unclothed. The parents also can subscribe to this, especially the mum, to relax and unwind from the daily chaos. A whole chapter is devoted later to promote the health of mother and partner, as an intricate aspect of relationship rebuilding or an antidote to stress. In addition, this exercise could reinforce the parents' relationship beyond the early days associated with the arrival of a newborn baby. The adjustment needed in this period could be a simple one, in the household.

Baby Massage, Its Definition?

'Baby massage' means gently rubbing and strengthening the arms and legs in a fashion that will cause no harm, and that is useful to the baby. It is essential to learn the methods before the birth of the baby, to ensure proper application when required. It is necessary for parents to master these methods of massage, which may prove valuable and worthwhile.

The definition according to Segen's Medical dictionary *(2014)*, denoting "a general term for the stroking of an infant by a parent or caregiver", with or without the use of oil. It is believed, that stroking often help to strengthen and regulate gastrointestinal and cardiorespiratory activity, relieve stress, tone muscles and relax the infant *(Segen's Medical Dictionary; 2012)*.

The Origin and History of 'Rubdown'

Whilst, hygiene, is at the core of this procedure, the expression 'Cleanliness is next to godliness'; has no base in religion. Although it is an old proverb found in Babylonian and Hebrew religious tracts, it is not in the Bible in this context. However, its debut in the English language found, in a modified form, in the writings of philosopher and scientist Sir Francis Bacon. He wrote in *Advancement of Learning* (1605), 'Cleanness of body was ever deemed to proceed from a due reverence to God.' However, nearly two hundred years later (1791), John Wesley referred to the expression in one of his sermons in the form we now use it today. He wrote, 'Slovenliness is no part of religion. Cleanliness is indeed next to godliness.' Personal hygiene and tidiness have nothing to do with holiness or godliness – the latter requires purification of the heart and soul to obtain.

The origin of newborn baby rubdown or massage is Africa, the perceived origin of humankind. However, the exact location of this practice though obscured, but acknowledged greatly, by the West African society. The idea of human water-birth was controversial, not too many years ago, but the demand is increasing now. This mode of birth, clinically, was undocumented prior to the current trend in healthcare practises in many countries, including the United Kingdom and the United States. However, now it is no longer a danger to the baby and mum, provided the carers maintain adequate care during labour and delivery. Moreover, in many healthcare establishments, their policy on water-birth, dictates the enrolment of uncomplicated pregnancies for water-birth. This mode of birth has since evolved, and it is now, heralded as one of the many natural birthing modes. Western history also indicates that the use of perfume was a practise common among the elites of many continents eons ago to mask smells, because some wealthy people in society washed infrequently, sometimes months apart.

So also is the newborn baby rubdown a likely source of controversy by many in the healthcare industry – until further study proves otherwise. This unique massage, though probably seen as controversial at the onset, is beneficial for newborn babies even beyond their adolescence, but the technique requires the parents and caregivers' approval. The quest to establish its origin and the acclaimed benefits began with a study. It is personally appealing to establish a scientific rationale in a social and global context of health research, together with ascertaining any benefits to baby. It would seem that the questions listed below are necessary, if to scratch the bare surface of this quest. These questions certainly deserve exploration and accord appropriate answers for impending users of the method.

- How safe is the newborn rubdown?
- Are the acclaimed benefits substantiated, specifically; the prevention of the malodorousness?
- Are the proposed products, approved for use on newborn babies?

These are examples of questions that parents and caregivers will ask. The study, conducted on a national level, received responses online from international sources, with questions ranging from any knowledge of the procedure and its origin in Africa to any concern with using or recommending newborn baby rubdown. In the overall sample of 203 respondents, the outcome and response were significantly higher than expected. The following people's graph summarised the result of the survey, with a significant percentage of respondents confirming their knowledge and origin of the newborn baby rubdown.

Squeaky Clean

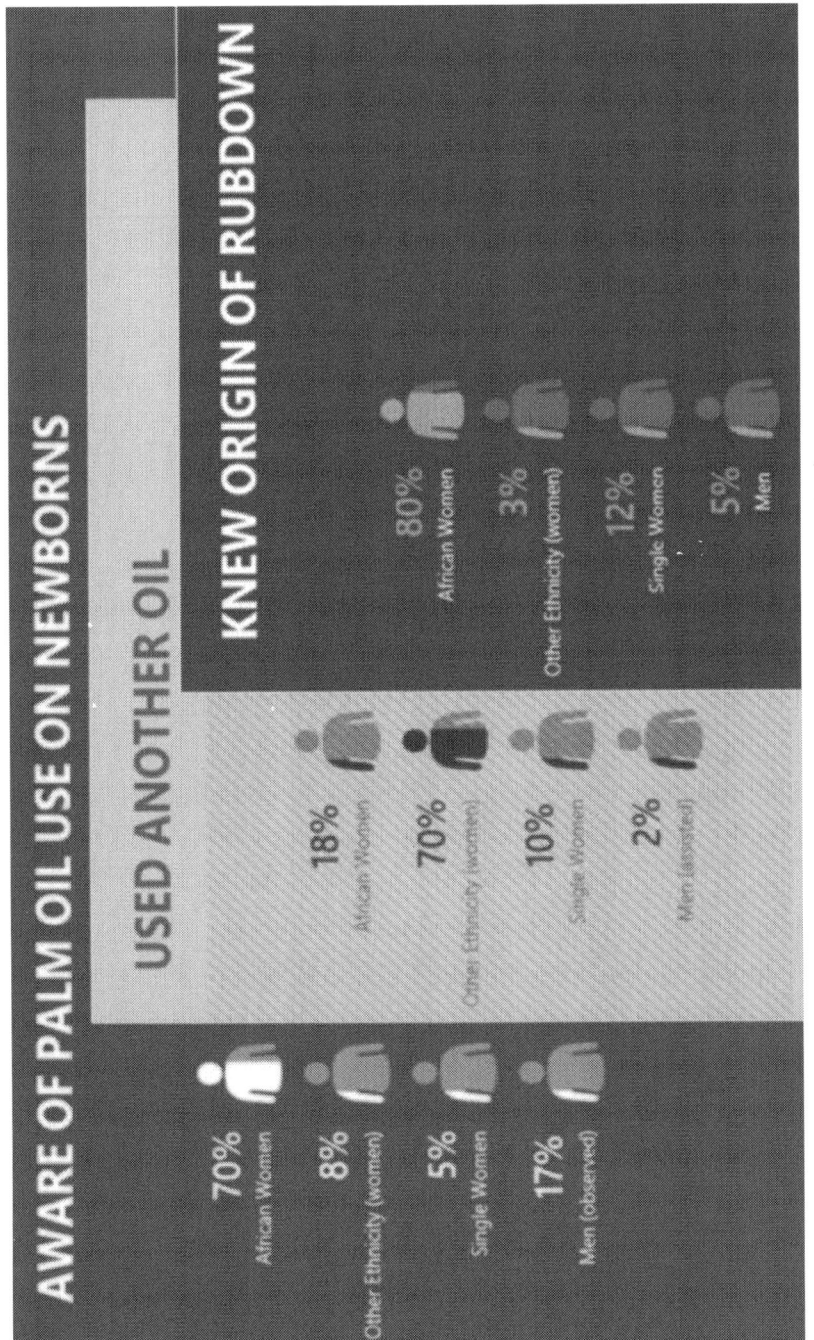

Survey of Palm oil use on Newborns

However, the greater number of respondents were people from African origins and with comments, such as, '...we gave our children this rubdown, but the same children may fail to apply it to their off-springs.' What is the reason? Their reason for this could be a lack of knowledge on the subject. The interesting bit, though, was the receptiveness of mothers surveyed on the streets of London. Some were surprised at the chosen oil, and some confirmed that although they have indeed heard about it, they used another oil such as olive oil. Because the alternative oil was neither due to the side effects of palm oil in its capacity to stain items, but the fact that olive oil was at hand. Sadly, enough, some African women were not aware of the procedure, and consequently they may fail to pass it on to the next generations. It is essential to give the younger generation the opportunity to acquire the knowledge, of an historic procedure such as, the newborn baby rubdown.

Do Newborn Rubdowns Differ from Infant Massage?

The rubdown is different from massage in its application and procedure. The gliding of the hands over the body of a newborn baby with the help of lubricant (such as red palm oil), and using very little friction without applying much pressure, is the definition of a baby rubdown. There was little reference of its (rubdown) definition though similar to infant massage, but differ nonetheless. However, the submission to include the word "baby rubdown" is sought with the *Oxford Dictionary*.

Whilst 'newborn' is medically defined as a baby at birth, and 'infant' is a baby from birth to year one, this definition may vary *(WHO 2013, Oxford Dictionary 2013, Beider S. et al., 2007, Hoath, Steven 2003)*. Furthermore, clinicians attest to using paediatric massage defined as complementary and alternative treatment of massage as therapy, or 'the manual manipulation of soft tissue intended to improve health and well-being' *(Vickers A. et al., 2004, Beider S. et al., 2007)* for children and adolescents.

Subsequently, infant massage is a complementary and alternative treatment that uses massage therapy for human infants. The practice of this therapy is evidently global for millennia and its use in the Western countries increases, as a treatment for infants, though some claim that the scientific evidence supporting its use is limited. On the other hand, parents see the immediate effect on the baby when used for ailments such as colic. However, research into the effectiveness of massage therapy on full-term infants has found some tentative evidence for benefits, such as restive sleep and less crying in infants. To base this procedure solely on clinical terms, will require more research to determine its efficacy. However, the benefits of the unique newborn baby rubdown appear in more detail in the later chapter. To draw one's conclusion solely on scientific research would gravely harm the future progress of humanity.

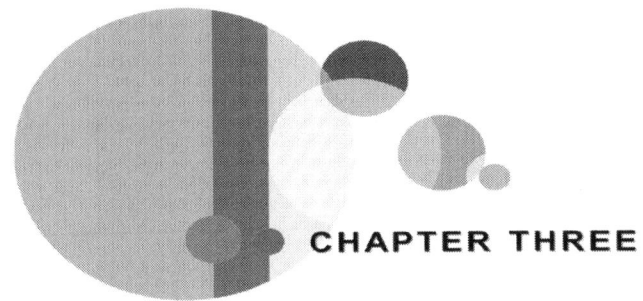

CHAPTER THREE

CLINICAL STUDY

To understand the full concept of the newborn baby rubdown and its credibility, a planned study ensued to investigate the effectiveness of the chosen oil-lubricant and its safety, as well as the safety of the rubdown and any adverse implications. There is no doubt that the unique newborn rubdown is special. The view of this procedure as controversial or radical and even old practise dragged into the twenty-first century with a twist in its application is understandable. There are previously minimal research base data of the effect of palm oil on microbes (germs or bacteria); however, none was present for the newborn baby rubdown. Consequently, any plan to implement a robust research is scientifically encouraged. Pioneering an idea based on ancient practises is not rare consequently, giving the technique the benefit of the doubt in any new or revolutionary concept; is seen as a progression perhaps, until it is, disproved otherwise.

The question, then, is whether it was speculative enough to warrant further studies, or whether it was just another clinical and commercial gimmick. A planned clinical study prior to publishing this book is considered prudent; to demonstrate the practicality of the method and to convey to parents the visual benefits seen immediately detailed in subsequent chapters.

The ideal focus will be on recruitment of parents from the anti-natal clinic, to demonstrate the method to them and subsequently provide support after labour and delivery. The study will take place over a specific time and within this period, to engage parents in subsequent massage technique and care. The number of participants will be relatively moderate compared to many scientific researches often carried out in clinical settings. It is my desire to use approximately two hundred babies for the study, specifically, to demonstrate the method. The goal of mastering the technique will not decrease. The idea will be to study the immediate effect of the process and subsequent questionnaire issued to record the experience from the mother's point of view, including the hands-on effect.

Research Methodology

The planned study of baby rubdown (controlled and randomised) using both quantitative and qualitative methods, firstly issued questionnaires for recruited parents. In the control group, the oil lubricant is red palm oil; rubbed on the whole body of the baby, avoiding the eyes. The randomised group will have a standard wash without the use of any oil (neither bleached nor deodorised substitute). Wherefore parents consented to the proposed study, they would neither be informed of their control or randomised assigned group; this is to disperse with any preconception before, during, and after the study.

Research Findings

The detailed result of this research is impending in the second (2nd) edition of this book, for clinicians, any caregiver and individuals who are remotely curious of the findings. The secondary result is no doubt pending in the light of the primary reason for the rubdown massage, which of course, is prevention of body odour beyond infancy. Malodorousness could take a long time to develop, and arresting this social impediment might prove essentially difficult, if unresolved. The outcome for this aspect of the study will need a long time for its verification. Nonetheless, it is achievable by only following the development of the baby, into adulthood. It is of course, a long waiting period, essentially, a dilemma for both clinicians and parents alike.

The formal and the latter, perhaps, experience the long-term effect or lack thereof of the secondary benefit, that is, elimination of body odour beyond infancy. The benefits observed primarily from experience following the process are outstanding by all accounts. These sensory observations as seen in chapter six of this book are:

- **Squeaky Clean**-the skin of the baby will feel clean, with memorable distinguish baby scent,
- **Sight-**the skin glowing, clean and radiantly so,
- **Touch**-feel the soft and smooth skin,
- **Restfulness**-baby will rest well quickly, falling asleep in no time. It is not a hoax, but visible and measurable facts and proof that parents deserve to know. The sheer joy of seeing all this is undoubtedly rewarding for all the invested energy, made by parents' and caregivers.

CHAPTER FOUR

WHEN TO GIVE A MASSAGE

The fusion of cultural hygiene (combined special newborn rubdown and first bath) and the modern practice of establishing and maintaining it is both practical and attainable. On one hand, very little effort is required to achieve the goal of cleanliness with a view to avoiding future body odour. Consequently, it is worthwhile to mention that this process will require mastering and carried out with the support of experienced practitioners. It is not a gimmick, and as such, parents acquiring the skill are privileged. They should seriously consider acquiring the skill and apply appropriately.

On the other hand, it is priceless, and time restricted; only at birth can, one achieved the full benefits of the massage and following bathing. It is senseless to avoid the use of this procedure for any non-credible reason. One surmised that any concerns were unfounded and reassured users to this effect, bearing in mind the careful research presented to alleviate any doubt in the method. If parents were in any doubt, then refer any concern to healthcare professionals. The procedure carries a minimum risk during the process provided one takes reasonable care to safeguard the baby.

The gravitas of this action has a lifelong impact on the confidence of the individual. Moreover, there is no known adverse side effect on the newborn baby if, the process subsequently incorporates the first bath following, this special and unique rubdown massage. To reassure everyone that if this technique of massage is tried, they will not regret it, but benefit greatly from it. Consequently, the advocacy of this technique is based on facts, with view to prevent malodorousness beyond childhood through, giving the newborn rubdown at birth or shortly thereafter. Why is this so? The answer is simple, to aid the general cleanliness of the body. In the quest to prevent body odour in infancy or beyond, it is recommended that the baby receives the benefit of the massage by its application at birth or shortly afterwards. This aspect, only applies to the first baby rubdown massage, which requires plenty of special lubricating oil. The massage method is different from the typical massages given to the baby. It requires steady hands and an experienced professional, and it guarantees to help the baby. There are also immediate and visual benefits such as clean, soft, and smooth skin. The other time that the baby may benefit from a good massage is a week afterwards. It is certainly a bonding exercise and event for parents to share with the baby. It is not to be taken lightly or for granted. The use of massage will enable the baby to settle, if feeling restless after a hectic day out from the uterus and into this big world. The experience of the new sounds, shapes, and smells later in life, as well as touch and many more, can be overwhelming for adults, and newborn babies are not immune to them.

Stress

Babies too can suffer from stress, just as much as adults can. In most cases, adults can take good care of themselves; this is not so for babies. Babies often express their emotions with cries or frequent fidgeting, and they rely totally on their caregiver, to provide for them. Note that not all cries are indication of stress or colic pain; however, there could also be an underlying cause, such as hunger or requiring a diaper change. Sometimes dealing with the symptoms of their crying can mask the cause of the problem; further investigation could reveal another severe cause in the first instant. It is worth further investigating; for example, contact your health professional. The other thing one needs to take into consideration is the aspect of any relevant experience. Ask yourself if you have dealt with the same symptoms previously, and how, it was safely resolve by the caregiver. If in doubt, call the experts – as mentioned earlier, better safe than sorry.

One of the possible methods to reduce colic pain in infants and new-borns is the application of a massage, which is clinically acceptable. The use of certain pharmacopeia should be a last resolve. The latter approach weighs heavily on medical consultation before use.

Colic

The *Oxford Dictionary*'s definition of colic is a form of pain that starts and stops abruptly. Baby colic, however, is a condition (usually in infants) characterised by incessant crying. This colic, also known as infantile colic, is a condition in which an otherwise healthy baby cries or displays symptoms of distress (cramping and moaning, to mention but a few) frequently, for extended periods, and without any discernible reason. The condition typically appears within the first month of life and usually disappears rather suddenly, before the baby is three to four months old, but it can last up to one year.

One study concludes that babies who are not breastfed are almost twice as likely to have colic *(Sung et al., 2014, cited in Roberts DM et al., 2004)*. The crying often increases during a particular time of the day, particularly the early evening. Symptoms may worsen soon after feeding, especially in babies that seldom belch. Always burp the baby after feeding; even taking water might require the parent to relieve the wind in the baby's tummy.

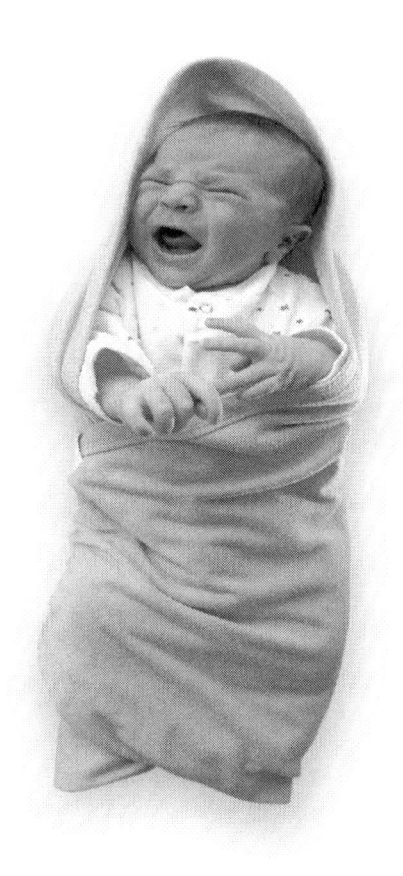

Crying Baby

    However, the strict medical definition of colic is a condition of a healthy baby in which it shows periods of intense, unexplained fussing and crying lasting more than three hours a day, more than three days a week, and for more than three weeks *(Barr, RG, Lust, Wessel, Saavedra, et al; 2003)*. However, doctors consider that definition, first described by Morris Wessel, to be overly narrow, and they would consider babies with sudden, severe, unexplained crying lasting less than three hours per day as having colic (so-called non-Wessel's colic). In reality, this extreme version of colic is more likely to be the final stage of a condition that has worsened for a few weeks.

Parents should seek help at all costs; preferably, medical assistance if this is the case with the baby. This is assuming the caregiver or mum has tried first massaging the tummy and then, if applicable, burping the baby. If the mother has practised this method with previous babies, then apply it. For first-time parents, do not be alarmed and endeavour to speak with a clinician. They can advise, and reassure one on the plan of action to take.

CHAPTER FIVE

BENEFITS OF THE UNIQUE NEWBORN RUBDOWN

The social ramifications of bad odour are unquantifiable personally, professionally, culturally, ethically, or otherwise. Although the baby will feel the immediate benefit of this special newborn baby rubdown, and to a certain degree, seen by the parents or the caregiver – it is indeed worthwhile. However, the benefits, of any massage, on either a baby or an adult, depend on the reason why it is given or required. Consequently, one's views the implication of opting out of this unique newborn baby rubdown massage may be seen, smelt, and even both. The former, however, moderately so, are seen immediately, and the latter may manifest years thereafter. The list below contain the most common benefits that are clinically proven, but are certainly not exhaustive:

- The proper application of newborn rubdown prevent malodorousness. This biomedical aspect led to the study described in chapter three. It is crucial to qualify this benefit in the light of its biomedical implication and to attain a credible reason for carrying out the procedure. It is for this very reason (proven biomedical reason in prevention of malodorousness) that this book is written for clinicians, parents, and aspiring parents. Though young adults may have had the procedure at birth, they were not aware of the methodology. For example, 85 percent of the women who completed the survey on newborn baby rubdown said; they do not know the reason why their parents used the technique. In addition to this, some respondents said it has been the traditional practice for generations. It is also important to note that though these babies are now growing or grown up, they are not aware of the traditional cultural bath given at birth. The general climate in Africa and the current global warming may play a role in the multiplication of bacteria on the body, leading to malodorousness. Overall, the elimination of this led to the concept and use of palm oil, which has cleansing and nourishing properties.

- Bathing will help the removal of vernix caseosa at birth, and as a result, the cultural fusion of the first newborn baby rubdown and the following bathing will ultimately aid hygiene. Whereas, the rubdown eliminates 100 per cent of vernix caseosa, bathing alone removes approximately 75–80 percent.

 The first massage of newborn babies locks in the moisture because many babies have very dry skin following birth. One could argue that all newborn have smooth skin, but this is not the case. As such, the great benefit of smooth skin will manifest from this simple procedure using the prescribed method.

- A softer skin texture will ensue following this process by protecting babies' delicate skin from the free radicals, also known as elements. The procedure of the first newborn baby rubdown and massage protects the newborn baby against dryness, as well.

- The massage can be relaxing for both mother and baby, seen as one of the special events for parents and child.

- A good sleeping regime will results in a better sleeping pattern and for longer periods. A daily massage of any form to aid the baby's sleeping pattern is inadvisable. However, a healthy baby – that is, a well-fed, cared, and loved child – will sleep regardless of a massage regime.

- Some believe that it has clinical benefits and children's hospitals often use the technique. Paediatric doctors recommend it to promote growth and development of preterm or low birth-weight infants, amongst other benefits cited in Vickers, A. et al., 2007.

- Massaging helps with wind (belching, releasing trap wind) and with many anti-climactic moments if the baby is not winding properly or at all. Apart from the baby vomiting all over himself or herself (even choking) or on the caregiver, there is also the likelihood of restlessness, wind, and colic pain.

- Many mothers can attest to using massage for colic relief. It was also a conclusive finding during the research and a well-documented benefit by all accounts.

The lists of the benefits are numerous, but let's not dwell on old folks' tales and pessimists; the goal is to educate respective minds. It is needless to force anyone to apply the technique, but willingly embrace it; in view of the child's social impediments that hinges on it.

In these modern times, research-based data is very vital and robustly encouraged in the health sector. It is no doubt standard and is vigorously recommended for advancement in many industries, especially healthcare. Innovation in any industrial sector is important for its progress, and not excluding the sheer opportunity of commercialisation. Consequently, the other useful reason for the research is peace of mind to caregivers. One cannot over emphasize the delicate nature of lawsuits against practitioners who ignore the safety of the baby in their care. In addition, to protect those who took adequate precautions during this process. It is the way forward, which is rigorously acceptable by the media and the public alike. This procedure is safe! Provided always, all due care is considered by the practitioners (clinicians, parents, relatives, and caregivers) to ensure the relevant guarantee from the experts in the industry. The level of care required is not different from other procedures carried out on babies.

CHAPTER SIX

HOW TO PERFORM A NEWBORN BABY RUBDOWN

> *In mastering the ultimate technique and the mystery behind the rubdown, also known as newborn massage, I assure you that it is a worthwhile investment and a very wise one at best.*

The newborn rubdown technique requires at least one observation of the method (or a practice on a doll) and attention is required particularly, to familiarise one with the anatomy of the baby. It will enable a smooth process for the rubdown. The image below is for illustration purposes only and not the exact likeness of babies. The body can secrete fluids with many functions, including lubrication of the joints to aid movement, saliva to aid mastication, tears to moisturise the eyes against free radicals, earwax to protect and clean ears, and vaginal fluid as a natural cleanser.

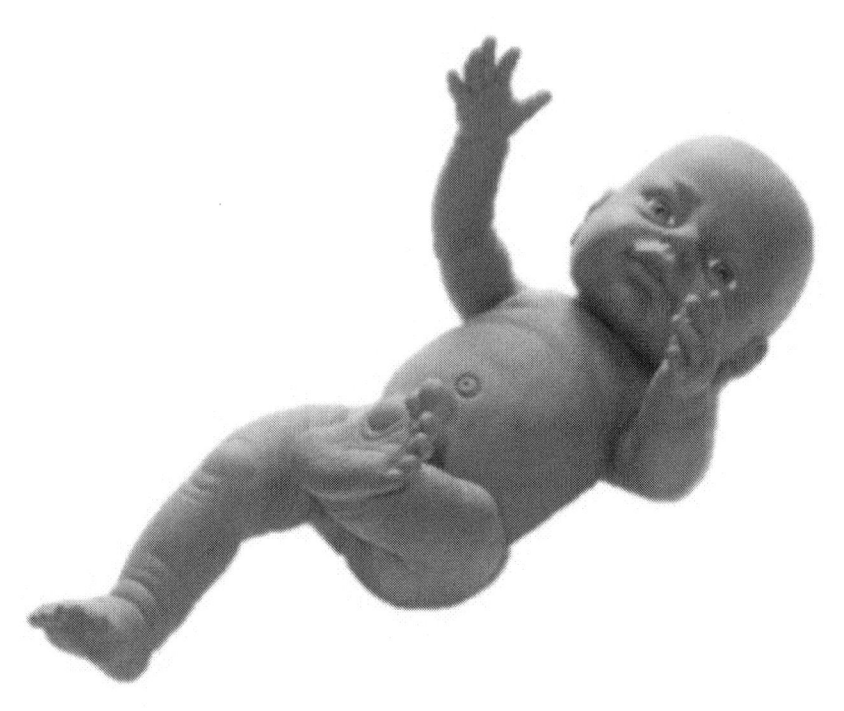

Baby Doll

So also is the role of vernix on the body of a newborn baby, to protect and reduce friction and aid in smooth vaginal delivery. The newborn baby usually covered with a substance called vernix caseosa, also known simply as vernix. It is a waxy or cheese-like, white substance found coating the skin of the newborn, and it is often sticky. Its full function is unknown. Its biological properties are to provide electrical isolation for the foetus, which is presumably an important aspect of developing foetal anatomy *(Saunders, C. 1948, Wakai, et al.; 2000).* In previous scientific studies, it showed an increased, evaporative heat loss in infants when it was removed soon after birth. However, newer reports confirm that washing the skin surface after birth reduces evaporative water losses compared to newborn with vernix left intact on the skin. Vernix caseosa is hydrophobic – that is, it is repelling, and it does not combine with, or is incapable of dissolving in, water (*cited in Wakai et al.; 2000*).

Vernix is theorized to serve several purposes, facilitating passage through the birth canal. It is slippery and thought to have an antibacterial effect; though there is little evidence to support a chemical role of vernix in protecting the infant from infection, it may form a physical barrier to the passage of bacteria that is in the womb, also cited in Wakai et al.; (2000). These functions are absolute and are no longer required following the birth of the newborn. Consequently, removing vernix by applying lubricant and subsequent bathing of the newborn is useful to maintaining the body temperature of the baby. The advocacy of the use of palm or olive oil at birth, to rid the baby of vernix is a tested, safe, and effective method. Preparation is crucial, as well as the actual application of lubricant in the rubdown on the baby and the following bathing. Please ensure that all bath time items required are nearby and ready for use.

Basic Items Required for Newborn Baby Rubdown

The items listed below are of preference to individual parents and are pertinent to this procedure. Replaced or altered these items with what is at hand. The special massage, however, dictates that the oil of choice be red palm oil roasted or cold pressed, and not deodorised or bleached or de-fractionised. The mother or caregiver will need a certain amount for the newborn rubdown. The purpose of recommending this oil is due to its properties and derivatives, detailed in the next page. In the event that the palm oil is unavailable proceed to use olive oil instead, either plain or virgin.

Mothers or caregivers may choose to sit on a low chair or the floor, or you may stand over a table; all positions are equally useful. A good recommendation posture is to stand for the duration, not only will it make the procedure quicker, but it is also efficient. Mother/caregivers, please make sure that, you are comfortable for this task. Do not rush into this procedure; great care is needed to accomplish the task while assimilating the experience for future use.

1. **Palm oil, 50–80 g, or 50–80 ml (ethically sourced)**

It may seem plentiful but is necessary to achieve the desired outcome. What is the point in using palm oil? Human use of oil palms may date as far back as five thousand years; in the late 1800s, archaeologists discovered a substance that they concluded was originally palm oil in a tomb at Abydos, dating back to 3000 BCE. They believed that Arab traders brought the oil palm to Egypt. The Palm oil plant *'Elaeis guineensis' is* mostly grown from the tropical regions of the world *(Kwasi P.; 2002, Reeves, et al.; 1979)*, it has long been recognized in West African countries and is widely used as cooking oil. European merchants trading with West Africa occasionally purchased palm oil for use as cooking oil in Europe. Palm oil became a highly sought-after commodity by British traders, for use as an industrial lubricant for machinery during Britain's Industrial Revolution including forming the basis of soap products.

It is semi-solid at room temperature; palm oil and palm kernel oil are among the world's most versatile raw materials. As a result, they are found in one or two supermarket products, ranging from margarine, cereals, crisps, sweets, and baked goods; to soaps, washing powders and cosmetics. Nevertheless, you may never have heard of palm oil since it is rarely listed as an ingredient on product labels, with the term 'vegetable oil' often being used instead. A regulation requiring the full listing of ingredients will soon come to force. Palm oil is also used in animal feedstuffs and as a bio fuel; this list is not exhaustive.

Squeaky Clean

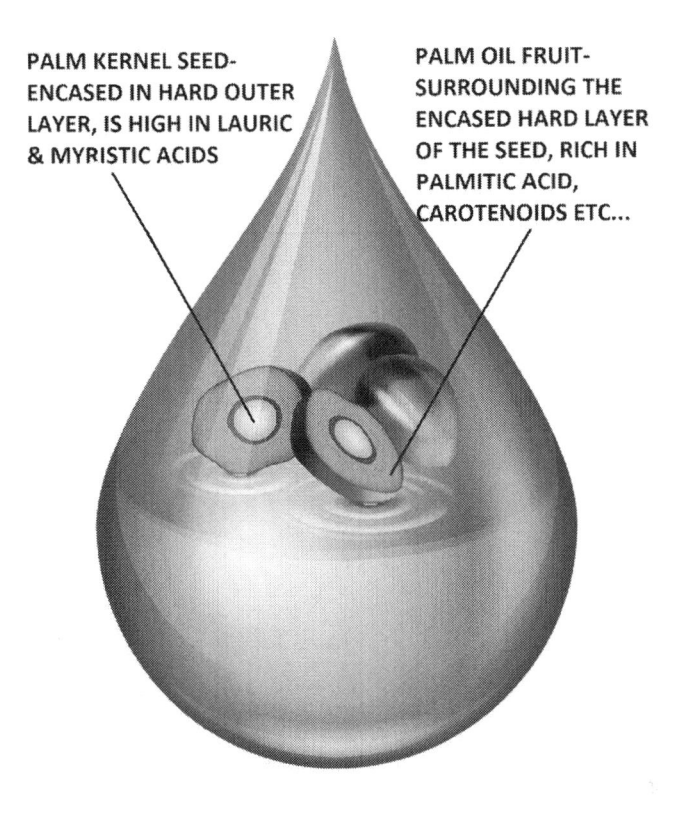

PALM KERNEL SEED- ENCASED IN HARD OUTER LAYER, IS HIGH IN LAURIC & MYRISTIC ACIDS

PALM OIL FRUIT- SURROUNDING THE ENCASED HARD LAYER OF THE SEED, RICH IN PALMITIC ACID, CAROTENOIDS ETC...

Palm oil Seed in an oil Droplet

Demystifying Palm Oil Derivatives

It is no mystery that approximately 60 percent of the palm oil consumed has been further processed into; a palm oil derivative or blend before incorporating it into the products we buy from the supermarkets. Having split into derivatives to produce a wide range of products, and as liquid palm olein (80 per cent) and solid palm stearin (20 per cent), it might then be blended with other oils, or undergo further processes to include interesterification, to create new oils with different physical and chemical characteristics. These derivatives sometimes used as ingredients, within shortenings, margarines for pastry and cakes, frying oils, coffee whitener, and emulsifiers. The act of further processing of the palm oil (purification) or simply bleaching it could influence the efficacy and further deplete its properties. Consequently, advocating using its pure form is highly recommended. Perhaps its pure form holds the mystery of acting against bacteria that causes odour and more. Research is yet to reveal this finding, but closer to home is the ability to cleanse, lubricate, and nourish.

Palm Oil in Wound Care

In a research study, there was no confirmation in the effectiveness of the use of palm oil to wounds for its supposed antimicrobial effects. Even so, there was a high degree of its effectiveness in some of the aspects in the tested microbes – a matter of fifty-fifty results *(Ekwenye U. N. et al., 2005)*. Oleochemicals are chemicals derived from plant and animal fats; they are analogous to petrochemicals derived from petroleum. (Are the Oleochemicals the bases for the odour eater?) Porim's scientists (Porim was renamed Malaysian Palm Oil Board in 2000) have long worked in oil palm tree breeding, palm oil nutrition, and possible oleochemicals use, in search of more uses of oil palm. Such is the versatility of this plant and its derivatives. The quest to confirm the derivatives responsible for eliminating odour continues, resources permitting, with the commissioning of an extensive study highly anticipated.

Red Palm Oil

Red palm oil gets its name from its characteristic rich dark red colour, which comes from carotenes, such as alpha-carotene, beta-carotene and lycopene, the same nutrients that give tomatoes, carrots and other fruits and vegetables their rich colours. It contains at least 10 other carotenes along with tocopherols and tocotrienols (members of the vitamin E family), CoQ10, phytosterols, and glycolipids. It is the practice to cold-pressed red palm oil since the mid-1990s and bottled for use as cooking oil, blended into mayonnaise and salad oil. Whereas, red palm oil antioxidants like tocotrienols and carotenes often added to foods and cosmetics for its health benefits.

A study in 2009 tested the emission rates of acrolein, a toxic and malodorous breakdown product from glycerol, from the deep-frying of potatoes in red palm, olive, and polyunsaturated sunflower oils.

The study found higher acrolein emission rates from the polyunsaturated sunflower oil (the scientists' characterized red palm oil as mono-unsaturated) and lower rates were observed from both palm and olive oils. The World Health Organization (WHO) established a tolerable oral acrolein intake of 7.5 mg/day per kilogram of body weight. Even subjecting palm oil to heat has proved that it is inconsequential as a mono-unsaturated in food. Subsequently, it is reassuring to know that it is equally safe for newborn babies in both its raw and refined forms, hence its use in body products (bath, lotions and shampoos) for even delicate skins such as a newborn. It could prove beyond doubt the save level for the proposed product, palm oil even in its raw state.

Refined, Bleached, Deodorized Palm Oil

"Various palm oil products are made using refining processes following milling, fractionation, and then melting and degumming to remove 'supposedly' impurities. The physical refining removes smells and coloration, to produce 'refined, bleached deodorized palm oil,' or RBDPO, and free sheer fatty acids, which are used in the manufacture of soaps, washing powder and other products. RBDPO is the basic oil product sold on the world's commodity markets, although many companies fractionate it further to produce palm olein for cooking oil, or process it into other products". (*Source: www.greenpalm.org 2014, Web 2014)*

> ***Note:***
> *There are variations between red palm oil and palm kernel; this includes colour, derivatives, and chemical properties.*

The following diagram and the subsequent one, illustrates many uses of palm oil and its by-products in infographic layouts. Whilst, the use of palm leafs in weaving products including, baskets, hats, bags, storage boxes and many more are common in regions that grows palm oil plant. The trunk of the plant are also useful as building material, with a capacity to provide a strong structure for traditional houses. The goal is to secure the trunk in clay thereby imbedding it into the structure, traditional builders have not departed from these custom. Whilst the waste products such as the shell from the seed (following extraction of palm oil) and other outer coatings are sometimes use for fuel, as much as the other parts of the plant, even, the trunk. These practises are common in the rural areas and alternative to stoves for camping in the forest.

Printable versions of these infographics are downloadable through digital platform. Copyrighted, all rights reserved, not for commercial distribution. Only one download allowed from digital version of Squeaky Clean eBook.

Squeaky Clean

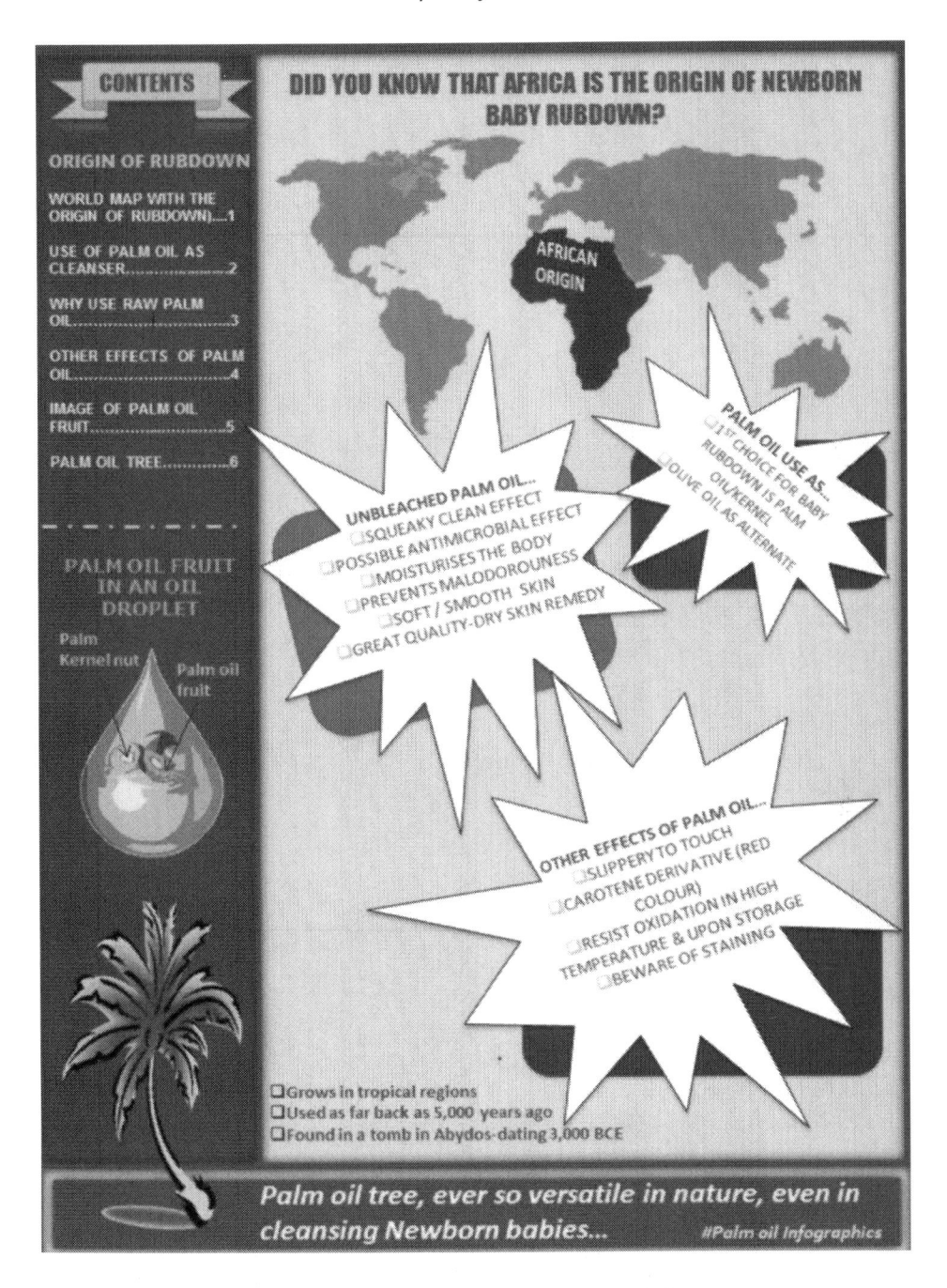

The Origin of Palm oil Use in Newborn Rubdown

PALM OIL USE & PROPERTIES
(Elaeis Guineensis plant)

- Rich red in colour,
- Rich in Vitamins A, E and minerals PERTINENT to SKIN repair,
- Very versatile use raw or fractionised,
- Lubricant in Newborn rubdown
- Found in food products i.e. baked foods, margarine etc...
- Use in cooking, frying,
- Use in cosmetics, i.e. soaps, lotions, creams etc...
- Animal feeds,
- Shell use for fuel,
- Weaving baskets, hats, bags, storage boxes &
- Building material, mixed with sand and clay.

PALM OIL AND WHAT THE PEOPLE SAID !

NEWBORN BABY RUBDOWN

...long hidden from the world the simple and cost effective way of preventing Malodorousness, from birth to adulthood. How is it done?

...such is the versatility of Palm oil tree!

The exact origin was believed to be in Africa and often practised by many, then passed on to the next generations.

...ethically sourced for newborn baby rubdown
...68% of women in recent survey either used it nor heard about it.
...80% of young people have no knowledge of it or its origin
...70% will use it if practical help is available
...20% used similar vegetable oil

SURVEY OF PALM OIL USE ON NEWBORN BABY

	African Women	Other Ethnicities	Single Women	Men (Mixed)
Used Palm oil/Aware	70%	8%	5%	17%
Used other oil/Aware	18%	70%	10%	2%
Knew Origin of Rubdown	80%	3%	12%	5%

Use a small handful of palm oil to fully cleanse the Newborn baby, then wash off ...

#Palm oil Infographics

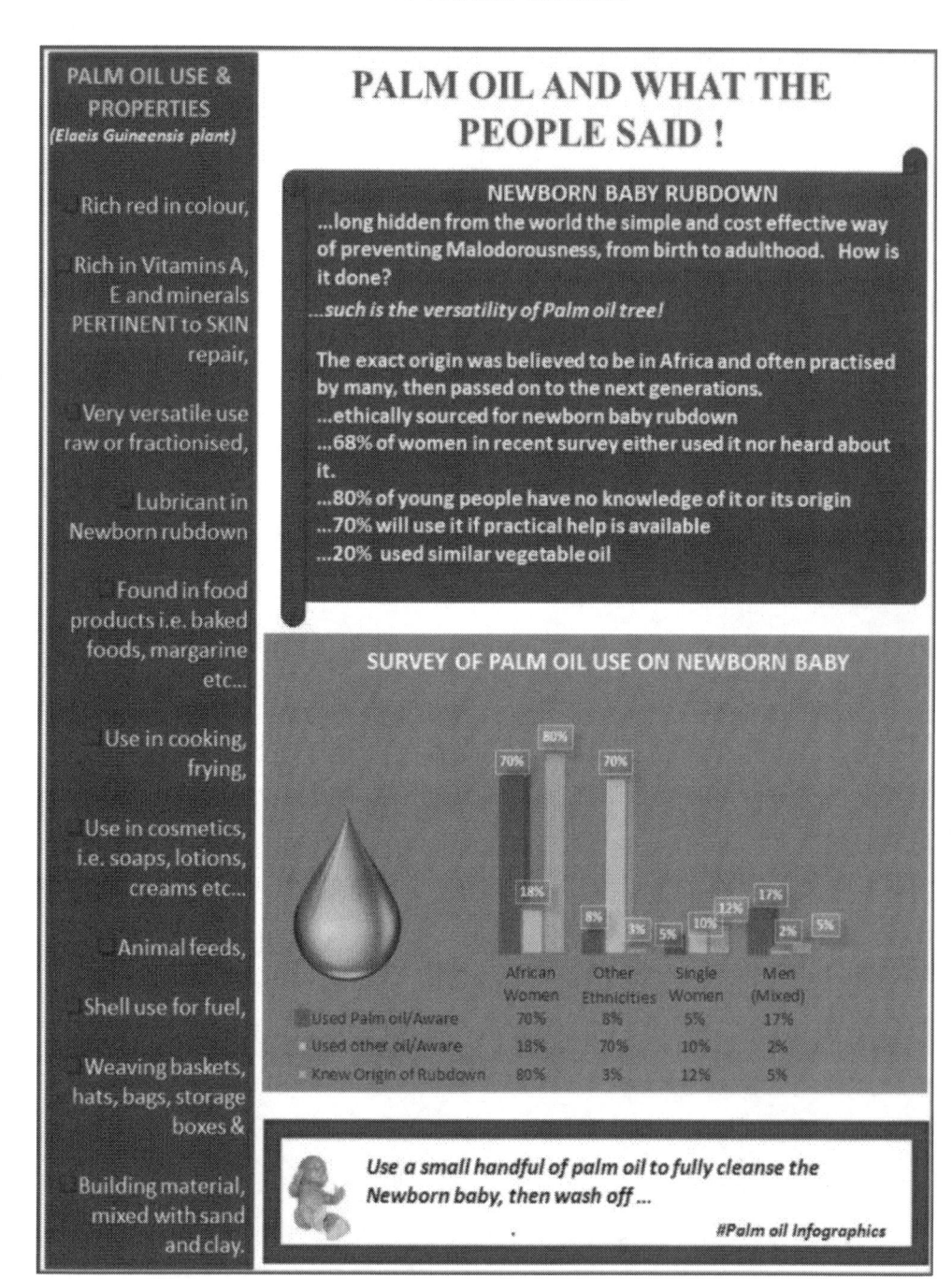

Palm oil in foods and use of its by-products

2. The second recommended lubricant is palm kernel oil 50–80 ml, derived from the innermost core of the palm seed. One of its characteristic features is the white colour similar to hard coconut, but it is not hollow.

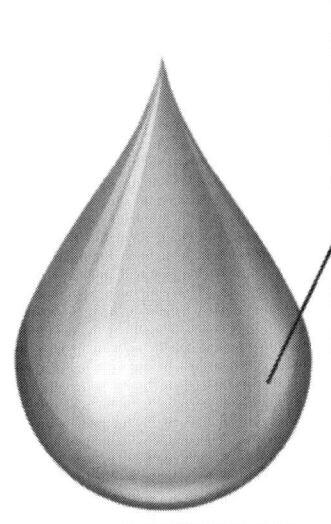

PALM KERNEL OIL IS RICH IN GOLDEN COLOUR-A NUT PRODUCT, RICH IN VITAMINS & MINERALS- MYRISTIC, LAURIC FATTY ACIDS, CALCIUM, MAG, IRON ETC...

Drip Palm kernel oil

It is a nut product, and great care should be taken by caregivers to avoid possible allergic reaction. In addition, refined oil from the palm kernel is often being used in beauty products. It is another form of lubricating oil that is used for the rubdown procedure. Although olive oil is an alternative, the recommendation of red palm oil is the first choice.

3. Clean flannel (washed at least twice before using on the baby),
4. Warm water to wash hands (you need warm hands to massage the baby, or simply rub your hands together after washing them) in a jug or bowl,

5. A baby sheet to place over the baby-changing mat or mackintosh is essential. It is a messy procedure, and as such, there may be staining of the clothing used. Use an old towel for the surface or over the mat,
6. A disposable sheet to cover the surface; this is another alternative to the baby sheet,
7. Bowl (basin or baby bathtub) to wash a newborn baby following, the use of the lubricant. Please note that the use of baby tub are for babies slightly older and reserved for much later,
8. All the bathing items – for example, changing clothes, towel, blanket, vest, jog suit,
9. Baby wash (natural or non-scented),
10. Cotton wools and balls (wool for the eye area and balls for the outer ear and nose areas),
11. Changing mat (to place on a flat surface or table); use in undressing, lubricating, and dressing baby,
12. Body lotion for after bath,
13. Plain sheet of cloth.

The table below list a guide to the main benefits of the preferred oil in the newborn rubdown. What are the reasons behind the cosmetic industry using palm oil and its derivatives in products such as soap, lotions, and body and hair creams? This product (palm oil and derivatives) contains many benefits for human beings, including hygiene. In its raw form (palm oil), the red colour has a tendency to stain and is messy at best. Nevertheless, these qualities are the only side effects on record, and this will not stop its versatile quality as a natural product. The benefits include its ability to soothe, lubricate, moisturise, and have a highly cleansing properties (its ability to dispense with malodorous from bacteria), amongst others. The probability of the latter, though unspecific, is a fifty-fifty chance, as indicated in the microbial study mentioned earlier. Although a versatile product to a level, it is still a hidden treasure from the wider society. The leading companies in the food, beauty, and toiletry' industrial sector use this product but seldom mention it. Perhaps if one cares to check the names of the contents of any product of toiletries currently sold in the market – items such as sodium palmate, sodium palm, kernelate palm acid, palm kernel acid, and tocopheryl acetate – a derivative of palm oil is most likely in them.

Benefits: Minerals and Vitamin in Lubricants

Product Name	Vitamins	Benefits
Red Palm Oil	Vitamin E	Renew skin, dry skin remedy, lock in moisture, help to prevent skin from ultraviolet rays
	Vitamin A	Repair, growth, and cell development; maintenance of the immune system and good vision
	Minerals	Completely free of cholesterol when ingested, other benefits not directly linked to its application on the body are its resistant to oxidation under high cooking temperature and upon storage
Side Effects		The strong carotene in the red palm oil has a tendency to stain surfaces or clothing, and it is very slippery
Palm Kernel Oil	Vitamin E	Renew skin, dry skin remedy, lock in moisture, help to prevent skin from ultraviolet rays
	Vitamin K	An essential fat-soluble vitamin that is important in bone health and as a coagulation factor in the blood
	Minerals	High phosphorus, calcium, magnesium, iron, and zinc; myristic and lauric fatty acids; suitable for the manufacture of soaps
Side Effects		None found, however it is a product of nuts of palm kernel, so possible allergic reaction; very slippery
Processed Palm Oil (processed, bleached, deodorised)	Vitamin E	Renew skin, dry skin remedy; lock in moisture. help to prevent skin from ultraviolet rays
	Vitamin A	Repair, growth. and cell development
	Minerals	Similar to the red palm oil in its original state, with reduced benefits of its minerals
Side Effects		Chemically processed with reduced benefits, and slippery

Squeaky Clean

Method Use in Newborn Rubdown

The waiting is over, it is an experience no doubt unlike any other. This technique exploits rubbing by sliding hands over the exposed surface of the baby's body without any force or application of pressure.

There are certain things that one will need to do first before engaging in the task. Make sure that all the necessary preparations, such as the required items are at convenient locations (arm's length away), ensuring that the room is adequately warm and bright, and an extra pair of hands, which is highly recommended for safety and dexterity. Often there is no shortage of people milling around newborns, so be sure to accept help from others.

> *Important Tips*
> *Handle baby with care at all times, especially during application of the lubricant. All lubricants are slippery; please take care when transferring the baby from the worktop or changing mat to the bath. The flannel will come in handy to pick up the baby safely and securely, place them into the bathtub.*

Newborn Rubdown & Bath

STEP BY STEP GUIDE TO NEWBORN BABY RUBDOWN

- Hold the baby's head with your left hand and use your right hand to apply the lubricant of choose
- Starting with the neck area of the baby, working your way downwards
- Apply to the neck, truck in a circular motion- pay attention to folds
- Hold each arm (one at a time) and apply from the top of the arm to the tip
- And do this again in a reverse order to the arms
- Apply the same method to the legs-but from the tip of the legs to the groin area - reverse and do it again
- Turn the baby around on their tummy mimicking sleeping position
- In the sitting position however, support the baby's head with your left hand
- Apply oil generously and massaging in an up-ward motion
- Gently rub it on the head of the baby, avoiding the eye area at all cost
- Cover the whole body completely, move to the ears, face and chin areas
- Place the baby in the water tub
- Washing the hair/head lastly

1. Choose the lubricating oil you prefer to use on the baby
2. Apply lubricant all over the body
3. Wash off with soap & water

Demo of Rubdown

Squeaky Clean

- Undress baby completely in a warm room (approximately 24 degree Centigrade),
- Choose the preferred lubricating oil to use on the baby,
- Apply the lubricant with bare hands previously warmed up or use a fine flannel for the groins and joints areas,

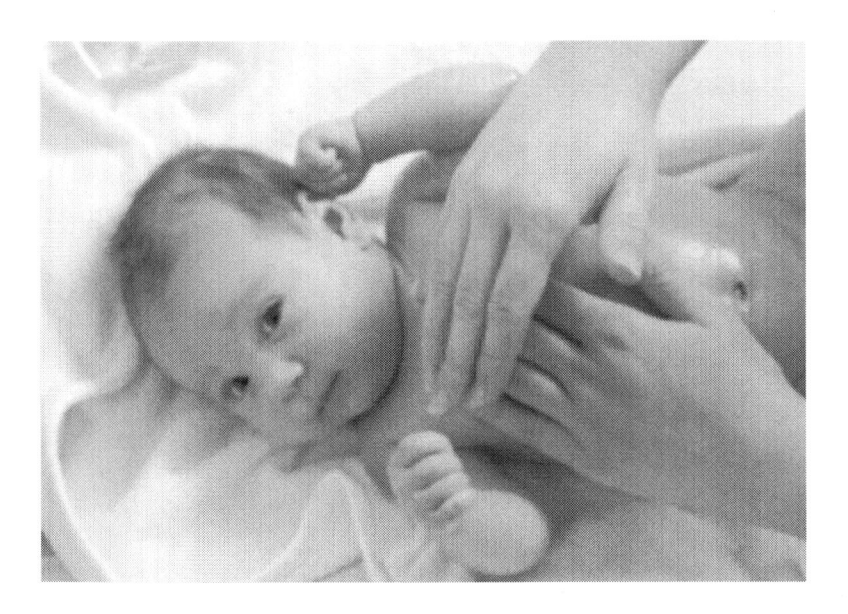

Application of lubricant on Baby

- Start with the neck area of the baby and work your way downwards,
- Apply to the neck and trunk of the baby in a circular motion, taking particular attention to the armpits and the groin,
- Hold each arm (one at a time) and apply from the top of the arm to the tip,
- Do the arms again in the opposite direction,
- Apply the same method to the legs, but from the tip of the legs to the groin area. Then reverse the order and do it again,

- Turn the baby around, now sitting the baby on your lap or lying her or him on their tummy, mimicking a sleeping position,

- Remember, if sitting down, you can apply the oil with the baby on your lap; ensure that you cover your lap with an old towel or clean sheet,

- In the sitting position, support the baby's head with your left hand under her chin and apply the oil in a circular motion all over the back of the baby,

- Apply oil generously, taking special care not to injure her, and massage in an upward motion,

- Finish the application with the head of the baby,

- Hold the baby's head with your left hand and use your right hand to apply the lubricant,

- Apply a generous amount and gently rub it on the head of the baby, avoiding the eye area at all costs,

- Once the whole body is covered and complete, move to the ears, face, and chin areas.

Finally, ensure that you have someone to help you at all times to provide the support you will need during this task. It is compulsory and relevant in the light of health and safety.

Congratulations on a successful rubdown, the bathing of baby follows afterwards! It gets better with every practice.

CHAPTER SEVEN

IT'S BATH TIME

The first newborn bath may be daunting at best, and an experience that is unlike any before; it is certainly unique by design. It is essential to give the baby a bath following the application of the generous amount of the oil, massaged into its body using a circular motion and paying particular attention to the groin, folds of the skin, and other spots. Do remember that giving the baby a bath requires ensuring safety at all times. The skin will immediately feel moisturised, smoother, and softer. It is the only time the baby will need such a detailed massage. Do consider giving a sponge bath in the next few weeks, and then that can be replaced by a tub bath. Whilst the former may be supplemented by 'top and tail,' especially, in winter seasons, the latter is an acceptable form of hygienically maintaining the baby's cleanliness for the first few weeks.

In one's opinion, this massage and subsequent ones will help build the baby and parent relationship – it is your ultimate bonding exercise. At other times, cooing, singing, and talking to the baby often promote bonding. Babies, love the sound of their mother's voice and will thrive on your soft and gentle touch. The challenge to you, therefore, is to try it, or ask for the assistance of an experienced person to guide you through the process of newborn massage and bathing.

Getting Ready for Baby's First Bath

The first bath is special, and subsequently giving a sponge bath is normal in the ensuing weeks. Use a warm room with a flat surface

Squeaky Clean

(like a bathroom or kitchen counter), a changing table, or a bed. Cover the surface with a thick towel or a mackintosh. Maintain the room temperature to at least 24 degrees Celsius (75 degrees Fahrenheit), bearing in mind that babies are easily chilled. It is essential to ensure all assembled items are within reach, before, the massage and subsequent baby's bath.

> ***Important:***
> *Never leave your baby alone in a bath, not even for a moment. If you have to go to the phone, the oven, or anywhere else, get someone to do it or wait until you have finished the task with your baby.*

Essential Items for Bath

- *Baby shower gel/soap (recommendation: unscented and natural)*
- *Baby bath sponge or clean flannel (twice washed)*
- *Clean blanket or bath towel (a hooded one is recommended)*
- *Clean nappy*
- *Clean clothes*
- *Clean vest*
- *Warm water (not hot; test with your elbow)*
- *Blanket to swaddle baby after bath*
- *Body lotion (mild and unscented)*
- *Comb*
- *Oil for the head*
- *Cotton wool and buds*
- *Barrier cream for nappy areas*
- *A clean cloth/towel (old) to transfer slippery baby from worktop into baby tub*

The Bath

Now that the application of the lubricant on the newborn baby is completed, it is time to remove the oil with warm water and unscented baby soap. Gentle sponge baths are perfect for the first few weeks, until the umbilical cord falls off, and the navel heals completely. The following are the basics of bathing a baby, and the relevant steps should be taken to ensure the baby's safety.

- Apply the soap to the sponge or flannel with a little amount of water.
- Place the baby in the water tub, supporting his head with the left hand from behind the back of the neck in a slightly sitting position.
- Pick up the soapy sponge with the right hand.
- Apply the soap to the sponge or flannel with a little amount of water.
- When using a baby sponge or flannel ensure cleaning one area of the body at a time. Start behind the ears and then move to the neck, arms, and elbows, knees, and between fingers and toes. Pay particular attention to creases under the arms, behind the ears, and around the neck.
- Towards the end of bath time, wash the hair and head to avoid chilling the baby.

Hold the head with the left hand, and wash that area last. Whilst newborn babies do not have much hair, sponging the few hairs is acceptable. To avoid getting eyes wet, tip the head back just a little when washing and rinsing, until the baby is much older. There is no need for shampoo; just use water for subsequent sponge baths.

Wash a little girl's genitals from front to back. If there is a little vaginal discharge, do not worry – and do not try to wipe it all away. If a little boy is uncircumcised, leave the foreskin alone. If circumcised, do not wash the head of the penis until it has healed. Splash water on the area when the dressing is off, and when it heals, wash with water and soap.

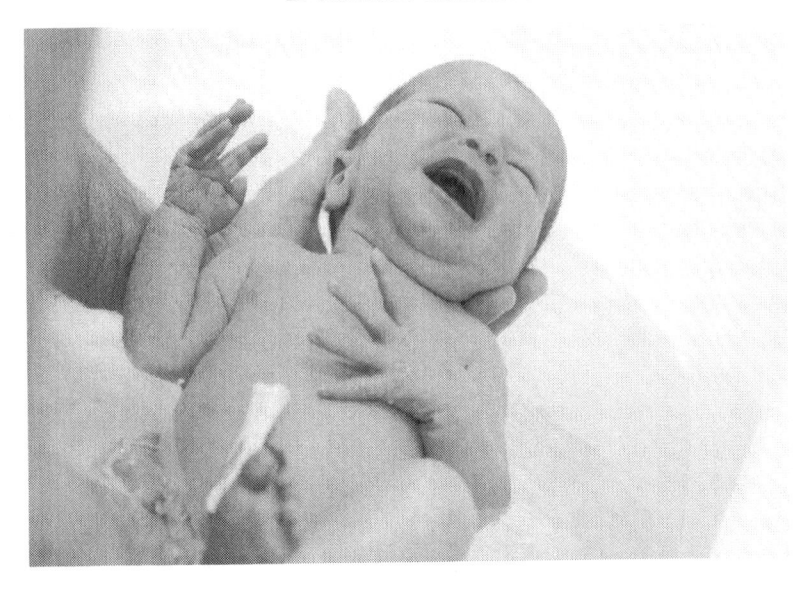

Bathing Newborn baby with cord clamp

- Using plain water or a mild, unperfumed soap, clean around the umbilical stump, this will only apply to subsequent baths (excluding the first bath, where an individual needs soap or shower gel; to remove the oil used during the massage). Once finished, wrap the baby in a towel and gently pat the baby dry. Rubbing the skin will irritate it and could lead to red skin or rashes.

Now that you have given your baby a rubdown and the first bath, proceed to dress the baby in the chosen clothes and feed the baby immediately.

> ***Important:***
> *You can apply the soapy sponge on the mat and transfer baby to the tub using the flannels.*

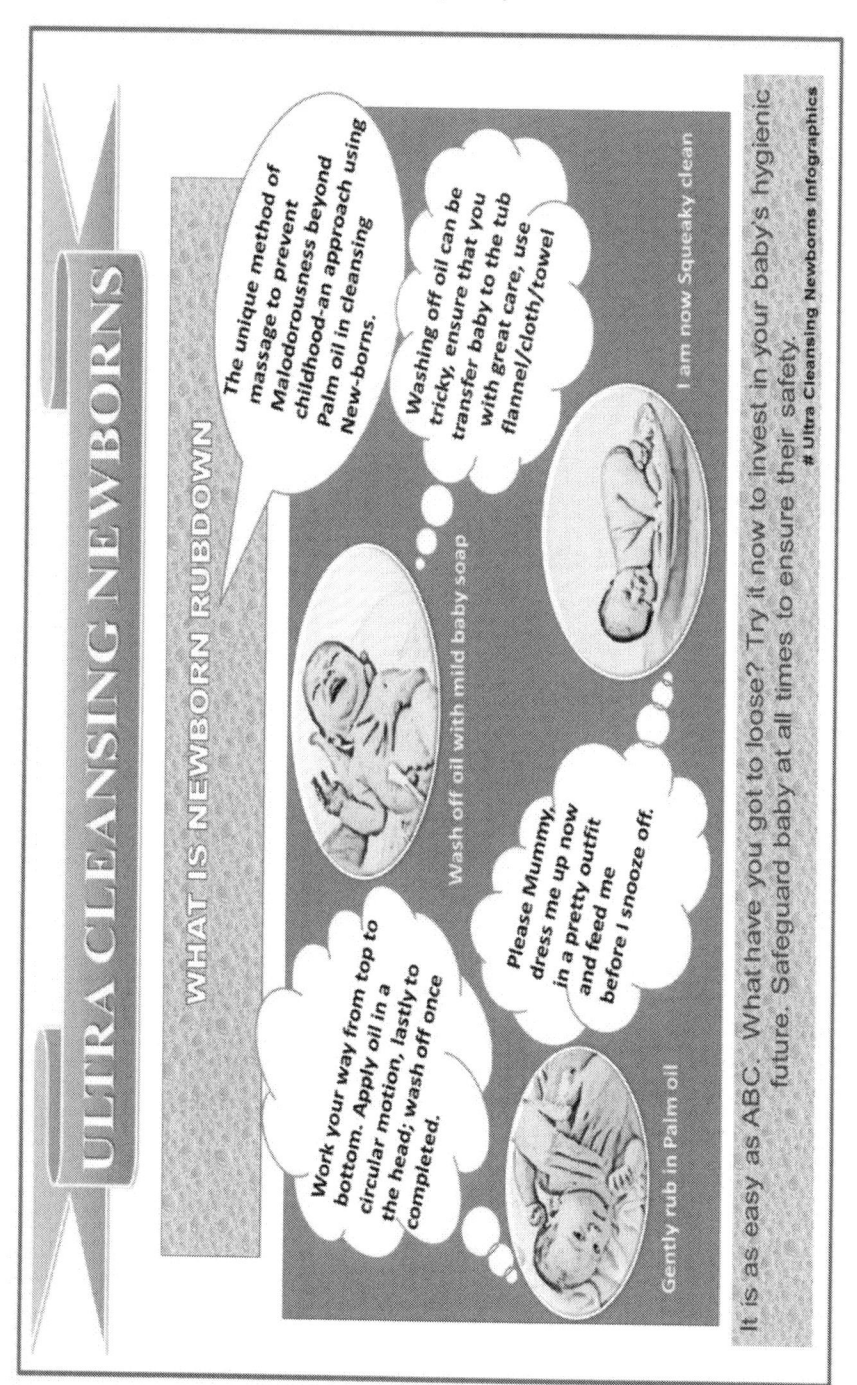

Squeaky Clean

ULTRA CLEANSING NEWBORNS

WHAT IS NEWBORN RUBDOWN

The unique method of massage to prevent Malodorousness beyond childhood-an approach using Palm oil in cleansing New-borns.

Washing off oil can be tricky, ensure that you transfer baby to the tub with great care, use flannel/cloth/towel

I am now Squeaky clean

Wash off oil with mild baby soap

Please Mummy, dress me up now in a pretty outfit and feed me before I snooze off.

Work your way from top to bottom. Apply oil in a circular motion, lastly to the head; wash off once completed.

Gently rub in Palm oil

It is as easy as ABC. What have you got to loose? Try it now to invest in your baby's hygienic future. Safeguard baby at all times to ensure their safety.

Ultra Cleansing Newborns Infographics

Ultra Cleansing Newborns-Infographics

The race to feed the baby is on because most babies will sleep for a long time after any massage. In addition, newborns are usually long sleepers for the first few weeks. Consequently, feeding the baby is as essential as giving the bath itself and will keep the baby hydrated. Tidying up can wait until after the baby has fed and been put to sleep. Remember to burp the baby after feeding.

> *Congratulations! Your little darling just had his or her first newborn bath. Your clean baby is ready for a clean nappy and clothes! Dress up the baby appropriately and proceed to feed him or her, as the baby is likely to nod off to sleep.*

Bathtub Time for Baby

In the subsequent months, the baby will require a different method of bathing that is less complicated and could be fun, as well. Give the baby sponge baths for the first month or so, until the umbilical cord falls off, the circumcision heals, and the navel heals completely. Thereafter, it is time to try to use the bathtub. It is understandable that not all babies will like the transition, so if the baby protests, go back to sponge baths for another week or so before trying again. Bathing a baby is a process; the adjustment required for both baby and parent is inevitable and should be approach with an anticipated learning curve. It is important to disperse with any anxiety for a better outcome.

Squeaky Clean

To Prepare

- Select a baby bathtub made of thick plastic and the right size for the baby. An insert for young babies is ideal; keep the baby's head out of the water. A slip-resistant backing on the tub will keep it from moving during bath time.
- Do not try to use bath seats or bath rings; these are for older babies who can sit up on their own, not for newborn babies.
- Make the first tub baths quick to avoid resistance and chills.
- Fill the tub with only two or three inches of warm (not hot) water; test the temperature with the elbow.
- Slowly lower the baby into the tub. Use one hand to support the baby's head at all times.
- Using a flannel or baby bath sponge, wash the face and hair last.
- When rinsing, protect the baby's eyes with a hand across the forehead; this is for older babies.
- Avoid soap on the face for new-borns at all costs, only use soap on infants if you are confident.
- Gently wash the rest of the baby with water and a small amount of baby wash.
- Use cleanser, wash, or water for hair. As the hair grows, try gentle baby shampoo.
- To keep the baby warm during the bath, cup (your) hand to let handfuls of water wash over the chest.
- Gently dry the baby by patting. Apply baby lotion all over to seal in moisture.
- Apply baby oil on the head of the baby if you prefer; brush hair appropriately. Please note that some babies' hair may not need brushing due to a lack of it.

Now it is time for a clean nappy. Apply nappy cream (barrier) to protect against irritation. When the bath is over, wrap the baby in a towel straight away, covering the baby's head for warmth. It is time to dress baby appropriately for the season and occasion.

CHAPTER EIGHT

SUBSEQUENT BABY MASSAGE

> *Important:*
> *When caring for a baby, think safety at all times to safeguard them. They are fully dependant on their caregivers.*

The discussion in the previous chapters contains a detailed process use in the unique newborn massage, together with subsequent bath to remove the lubricant. Although, mentioned subsequently is the baby massage for therapeutic purposes, they are not in chronological order to emphasise the absence of similarity of both massages. This chapter is devoted to teaching the method used in subsequent baby massages. Due to the delicate and fragile nature of babies' anatomy, the methods of massage accorded to babies are of gentleness and without pressure. To achieve this, avoid causing direct or indirect injuries to the baby.

It is necessary to take adequate care to safeguard the baby against any injury. Remember, the purpose of the massage is to relax the baby, avoid pain or any agitation to any injuries. It is equally important that the caregiver be relaxed to undertake the baby massage. Mothers that tried will attest to the benefits. Those

Please:

- *Use a warm room in winter*
- *Wash your hands*
- *Use warm hands (rub together if cold)*
- *Ensure the baby is comfortable*
- *Ensure the baby is not hungry (but be ready for another meal after massage)*
- *Ensure the baby is not sleepy*
- *Ensure the baby is not too tired*
- *Ensure the baby is not injured*
- *Ensure the baby is not sick and requiring medical aid*
- *Use suitable positions. Either sit on a clean floor or stand by the table. You can choose to use a baby changer on the table or the floor.*
- *Use a covered pillow with a clean sheet on the table, or a pillow covered with a sheet on the floor.*

prepared to try it should analyse the overall process and thereby provide feedback.

How does one avoid causing injuries during baby massage? Should one forgo this practice for the fear of causing injuries? The answer is no! In my opinion, finding a qualified healthcare practitioner (that is, a nurse, doctor, or a midwife) who has the knowledge to help with the process is prudent. There are many avenues of obtaining the required information to enable this process to go smoothly for the baby and for whoever performs it.

Try to get the attention of the baby (speaking, cooing, smiling,

> **Items Used for the Massage:**
>
> - *Palm kernel oil; avoid if baby is allergic to nuts*
> - *Mint oil*
> - *Camomile oil*
> - *Safflower oil*
> - *A clean flannel, to wipe away excess oil (there is no need to bathe the baby after this massage, provided baby is clean)*
> - *Warm water to wash hands*
> - *Warm water to dip flannel into following the massage*
> - *Bowl containing warm water*
> - *Changing mat, to place baby on during massage*

singing,) before proceeding with the task of massaging; this is a form of obtaining permission or consent. Grab the baby's attention, by talking in a quiet voice, and smiling at the same time. Please note that this latter part is not applicable to the newborn rubdown massage detailed in the previous chapters.

Although there is no research on whether asking for the baby's permission facilitates the process of massage, one can only assume that it is in the best interests of the baby to have this experience before the massage. In view of this, ask yourself whether talking to your baby is beneficial.

Although the method for the first massage requires the application of a vast amount of lubricating oil, the following one requires far less. Start with the trunk area (the chest and abdomen towards the groin area) and work your way down the arms and legs. There is no need to involve the head or apply oil on it. The best application is, with the baby turned on its back, is by using both hands. There is no need to involve the groin area and the armpits. To apply oil to the back, use the same method as above and turn the baby on its tummy. Do this by supporting the baby with the left hand and only using the right hand to apply the lubricating oil. However, older babies can completely lie down on their tummies. Repeat these steps three to five times on each aspect of the body, gently running the hands all over the body.

Finish up by holding the baby or supporting him in a sitting position (depending on his age). Take special attention and care at all times to avoid injuries, due to the fragility of the baby and the slipperiness of the oil. This massage, often given to babies who have had a bath and are clean, unlike the newborn massage, where it is compulsory to give a special bath afterwards. It is your choice to wipe off the oil with a flannel dipped in warm water when you have finished massaging.

Newborn Kits

A trunk box specifically for indoor is useful for the newborn. Mothers can choose to have a special one built. It is essential to invest in one that is durable with relevant items before the birth of the baby is advisable and essentially sensible. The items listed below are a guide; modify them as required. Putting these items together is easy, whether purchasing individual items or buying collectively as an investment. The materials for the trunk could be made of durable aluminium or wood and lined with fire-retardant fabrics; this can be passed on to the next generation of babies, a sensible 'hand-me-down' that is worth investing in for the baby. Often, refilling the trunk with newer items for the next baby is highly recommended. It is up to the parents to make the right decisions, so invest in a very good kit to use for the children.

The lists below are some of the items found in a pre-ordered baby trunk; these items and many more are included in many kits for newborn babies. The design of the trunk box is uniquely for indoor use, whilst the changing bags are for the outdoors and come with varying designs and sizes.

An Outdoor Bag with Baby's Essentials

The content of this bag is to ensure that essential items the baby requires when outdoor are readily available. However, items are in a much smaller quantity, for example, one or two extra clothing's, dippers, wipes and feeding items. This is just a guide, and parents can modify the items as needed.

Mother and Baby Unit

It is customary to provide a unit that the mother and the baby will benefit from in parenting. Consequently, the proposal of such a unit planned that merits the occasion and is environmentally robust enough to demonstrate the techniques for the newborn rubdown is anticipated. This unit is a centre where parents may drop in or come in for an appointment to master the methods of baby massaging. They participants are guaranteed interactive and stimulating activities. The support available would vary, and networking with other parents may be beneficial and invaluable, especially when it is the mother's first time. The experience of being in a group can provide many benefits and the opportunity to discuss and exchange ideas. Given that caring for a newborn baby is daunting at best, an engagement of expertise in many aspects is the norm, whilst others may come naturally (for instance, breastfeeding). These are some of the issues that one propose to discuss, tailored to individual needs, and reviewed periodically. The duplicity of the activities at the unit will be avoided to create uniqueness' compared to the present care provided by any group, health authority, or organisation.

Recommended Items in Baby Trunk Box:
- *Baby bath sponge*
- *Blanket, Bath towel (one hooded, one flat)*
- *Bed Sheet*
- *Baby food warmer*
- *Baby sponge*
- *Baby wipes*
- *Baby shampoo (×4)*
- *Baby shower gel (×4)*
- *Cotton buds (in lid-covered ceramic mug)*
- *Cotton wool in its jar*
- *Camomile oil / Mint oil / Safflower oil*
- *Comb*
- *Ceramic bowl*
- *Changing mat*
- *Feeding cups (×2)*
- *Feeding bottles (×2)*
- *Feeding dish, Feeding spoons*
- *Flannels (×10)*
- *Gauze*
- *Nappy (in cotton bag)*
- *Nappy disposable bags*
- *Palm kernel oil (×2)*
- *Shea / Cocoa butter*

CHAPTER NINE

ME TIME

The contents of this section embody a personal and professional experience, although leaning more, towards the former. This section and the following chapter is devoted solely to parents, who are stronger in the partnership of raising their children. To reaffirm the role of a woman in this wonderful time of pregnancy, delivery, and being a new mum, regardless of whether it is the first time or subsequent births. Can the arrival of a newborn in the house be any more exciting and delightful than this? The sweet, adorable face of the baby enthrals everyone, but there is more to the cuteness of the little bundle of joy, and new parents will have to do a whole lot of feeding, changing nappies, and putting the baby to sleep. All these can be demanding and chaotic for the entire family.

The baby will keep everyone on their toes with its constant cries for attention, wailing, drooling, and bumping into things, as it grows older. Parents may lose some sleep in trying to get the baby to settle, with life taking a huge turn once the baby arrives home.

The parent deserves pampering as well, especially, the new mum. Who is in the best position to do this for the mother, but a very able body, perhaps a–partner, or any close friend or family member? Mothers can bask in the moment and receive attention from all directions. It is no wonder some women tend to have babies every year for many years. However, the attention from relatives, friends, and one's partner can be overwhelming and too noisy for both baby and mother. One of the ways mothers can de-stress is relaxing by massage.

Squeaky Clean

An essential recommendation for mums', of a dose or two of good adult massage, this is indeed, an indulgence worth investing in, a tool in its own right. It is both a formal and informal form of relaxation or stress management after the whole process of giving birth, and often it helps with the early days of sleep disruptions.

The following infographics illustrates an affirmation of the state of the body when massaged. It is more capable and fit for any action, including, healing, relaxation, receptive, to mention but a few. In addition, the mind aspires to a relaxed state and a positive mind-set ensues, together with the spirit and soul in oneness with the body. It is an all-round balance of the body.

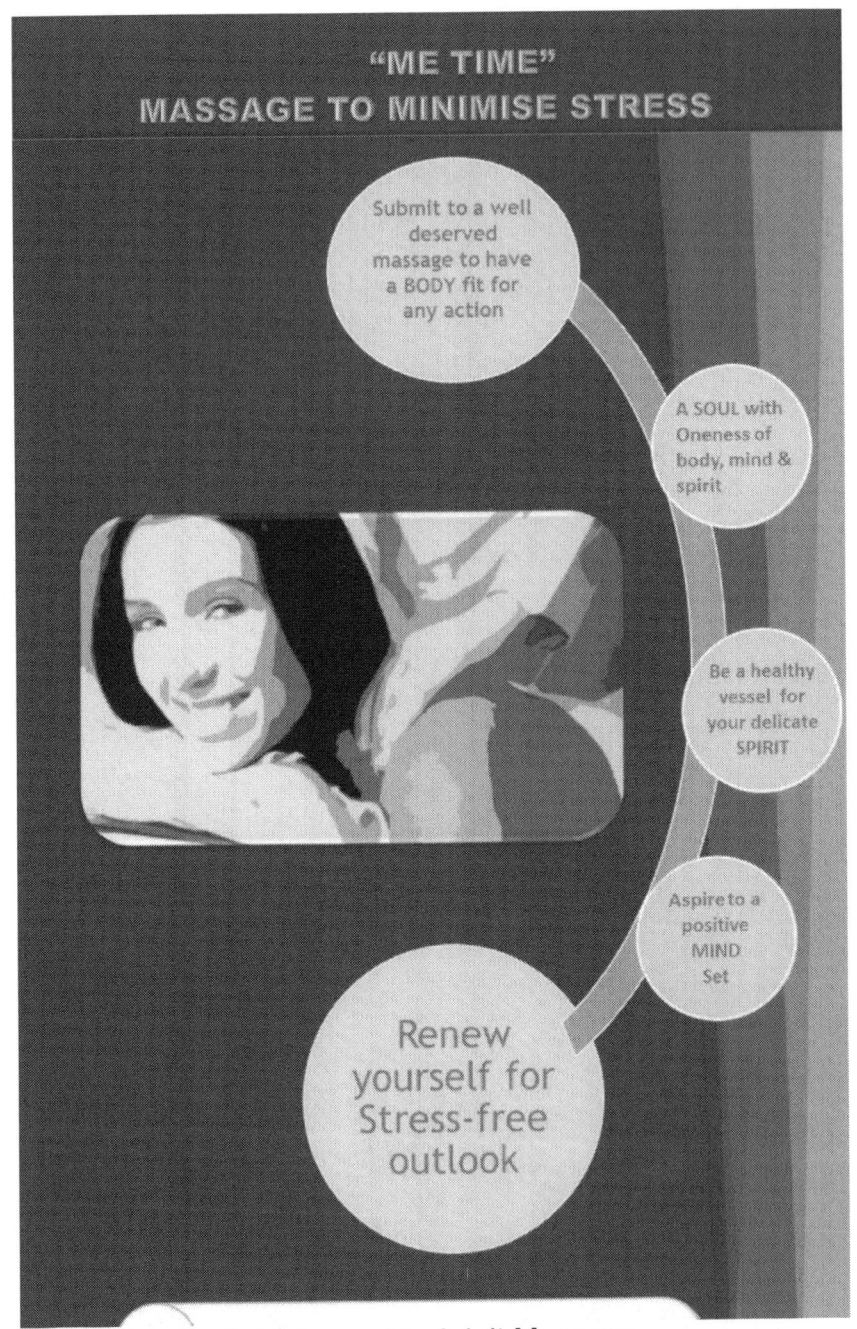

Part 1 infographic Adult Massage

This experience will also help with rebuilding one's relationship with their partner after the ordeal of labour, whether the birth was normal or instrumental (e.g., caesarean births). For the father there is no denying that the experience of massaging one's partner will be memorable, beyond releasing stress and the ultimate relaxation mentioned earlier. Whilst the process is similar to baby massage, more pressure is needed to loosen any tight muscular tissue on an adult. This massage is a style of touch that can be sensual or non-sensual, and it is very effective either way. Therefore, whichever direction the session takes, it is a good way of building (or rebuilding) physical trust between a mother and her partner, and it is a great opportunity to reaffirm each other's bodies in a safe yet intimate way. When the spouse gives mum the massage, both parties can decide what direction they desire the massage to take. Moreover, mothers should do this when they are comfortable enough setting their own boundaries.

This other option (beyond the shoulders) is sensual in its use and might be easier after the six-week post-delivery checks for mum and baby. It is up to one to determine the ceremony of preparing the location and lighting of scented candles is optional, which might be unwarranted at the initial exercise. Time permitting; one may choose to indulge a bit further. In view of this, just sitting on a chair or any other position, including lying down, is acceptable. Choose to be either fully or partially clothed, depending on the method the person uses and their mood. Sometimes there could be an opportunity to use massaging oil for the exercise.

In all circumstances, the goal is to benefit from the process of massaging and spending quality time with one's partner. In the event that the mother is not ready due to stitches, do not concern yourself on the missed opportunity – take your time and do it when you are ready. The opportunity to do full-body massage will present itself, and when it does, seize the moment.

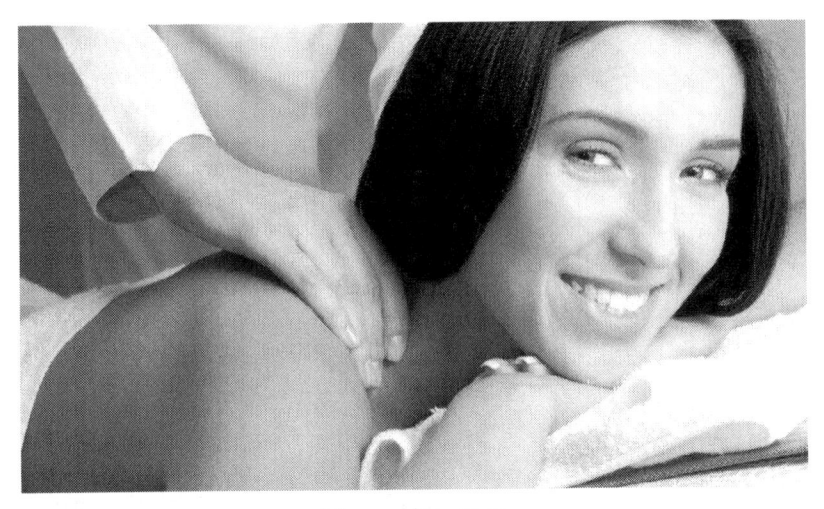

Massaging mum

The absence of stating the technique of adult massaging (both commercial and non-commercial) is intentional, to give couples the opportunity to discover for themselves what works and what does not. Either one discovers pleasurable points or angles during the process; it is all about the journey of discovery and its use thereafter. Do explore and discuss your feelings to build a stronger relationship.

In the meantime, proceed when ready with a basic adult massage, starting from the shoulders or the part of the body involved in lifting. Using a firm grip, rub from the neck area down to the shoulders.

The second part of the massage infographics illustration demonstrates the benefits and general tips of massage for inspirational purpose.

DID YOU KNOW THAT...

Resting will ensure that the Body recharges to embody a wholesome Soul that supports a healthy lifestyle. Whilst a troubled mind will pose a health risk, always think positively, for a burdened mind can readily break ones spirit and drain you physically, emotionally, mentally, financially...

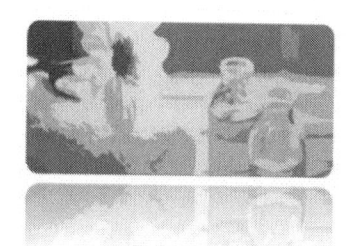

The true benefit of body massage cannot be fully quantified-however, many attested to the following listed BENEFITS:

- ❖ DEVELOPED BETTER SLEEP PATTERN
- ❖ HEALED FROM ACHES / JOINT PAINS
- ❖ CONCENTRATES BETTER ON DAILY TASKS
- ❖ BETTER MIND SET AND MORE RECEPTIVE
- ❖ INCREASED ENERGY
- ❖ HEIGHTENED SEXUAL APPETITES
- ❖ INCREASED OXYGEN TO THE BRAIN & OTHER TISSUES
- ❖ BETTER LYMPHATIC DRAINAGE
- ❖ VISIBLE GLOW TO THE SKIN
- ❖ RELAXED MUSCLES

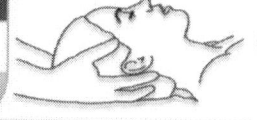

A recommendation of balanced diet, good intake of plenty water, loving care, exercise and rest, regular massage; it is all the mother requires towards a stress-free lifestyle.

IT IS NOT NECESSARY TO USE OIL OR ELABORATE SETTINGS FOR MASSAGE PRE OR POST DELIVERY. TRY SCENTED CANDLES. PARENTING MODE OUGHT NOT TO BE STRESSFUL-SET & AGREE YOUR BOUNDARIES AND PREPARE TO RELAX. ENJOY!!!

Part 2 - infographic Adult Massage

A recommendation of the application of massaging oil (scented or non-scented, olive oil, baby oil,) to avoid friction on the skin or parts of the body, but it is not compulsory. Should the 'mum' wish to switch and return the favour by reciprocating the process; your partner will handsomely reward it. It can facilitate couples rediscovering one another, and it is a very strong relationship tool endorsed by relationship counsellors.

Self-Massage

We all indulge in many forms of activities to improve our wellbeing and a regime of exercise and balance diet, together with good intake of fluid (water) will enhance one's immunity against diseases, towards a healthy lifestyle. Suffice to mention that not every mother will have someone else to offer her massage in her time of need. It is not uncommon, but do not despair at missing out on the benefits of massage. It would be wonderful if everyone has someone to give them a massage every day of their life, moreover, it takes time and money if one engage a practitioner. To give oneself a massage eliminates all those concerns mentioned above: it is cheap and can be done anytime or anywhere.

So WHY self-massage? The obvious things comes to mind, such as self-preservation and the countless benefits, including the following:

- Warms and relaxes the muscles,
- relieves tension,
- it helps to reduce stress,
- it increases the blood circulation,
- it increases lymphatic drainage,
- it helps to improve the immune system,
- it helps the body eliminate excess fluids,
- it lower the blood pressure,
- it tones the muscles,
- it tones the skin,
- it is a form of a passive workout for the body,
- it helps to eliminate waste products,

- it improves the flow of intestinal fluids, thereby improving the appearance of the skin, especially in areas prone to cellulite.

It is essential that the person be relaxed when carrying out self-massage, as one might need to work in some awkward positions and do not want to cause any twists or injuries. Endeavour to carry out all massage strokes towards the heart as this helps the passage of blood throughout the body and increases the circulation of both blood and lymphatic flow. It should be relaxing, warming and smooth soothing feeling and should not cause pain, though discomfort at times, but actual pain is improper. The massage stokes should work in time with ones breathing, not seemingly hyperventilation as some mothers engaged in at the process of labouring, but of a regular pace. Once the massage progresses and the muscles become warmer, the strokes can become more vigorous and intensify at will. This intensity will help to sort out deep-seated problems or tense muscle conditions, although, this is better achieve if one is receiving than self-application.

Self-Massage Techniques

It is a common knowledge that most standard massage stroke can be converted for self-massage, provided always, that one observe the general rules of massage. The technique entails directing the strokes towards the heart, pushing the blood around the system in conjunction with the circulation and not against it. The following points summarise the self-technique:

- The option to use body lotion or massage oil is really up to one, but its application will reduce friction, in turn causing no injuries or bruising.
- Either ensure to use the flat hand (fingers together, palm down) or the ends of the fingers (bunched together, please no fingernails).

- Work in an upwards way by first placing the tip of your right hand over your left hand. Gradually work way in an upward stroke and repeat the same with your left hand.
- Apply the same principle to your lower limbs and other parts of the body, three or five times.
- All massage stroke should start lightly and slowly build to a firmer more rapid pace.
- The body (flesh) should be warm and relaxed before using any deeper strokes, bear in mind that, working deeply on cold, tense flesh will feel unpleasant and cause bruising.
- The rule of massaging dictates that it should never be painful or sore, but massage that is too light is little better than a comforting stroke.

The process of undergoing a nine-month pregnancy and the ensuing labour might seem like a journey of a lifetime. In fact, at the end of this journey of pregnancy, labour and delivery, is the miracle of life and subsequently the beginning of another wonderful one. To care for a newborn ought not to be stressful, but there is a learning curve for both parents and eventually the baby. One can attest that the courage and overall spirit needed to care for a newborn is not magical and will not materialise from thin air. However, by learning and mastering the basic technique of care even, Newborn-rubdown, one becomes confident and proficient at the skill. Practise makes perfect and trust your maternal instinct!

CHAPTER TEN

STRESS LINKED TO BIRTH TRAUMA

"It is believed that between 25 and 34 percent of women report that their births were traumatic *(Soet J. E, et al., 2003)*. A birth is said to be traumatic when the person (mother, father, or another witness) believes the mother's or the baby's life was in danger, or that a serious threat to the mother's or the baby's physical or emotional integrity existed" *(K. Nicholls et al., 2007)*. Following the birth, some women go on to develop post-traumatic stress disorder (PTSD) or post-natal depression, a severe and long-lasting reaction to the trauma. The latter associated with birth and other organic factors. The diagnosis, based on the following criteria from *the American Psychiatric Association's Diagnostic and Statistical Manual of Mental Disorders, fourth edition*, with at least nine symptoms from the following categories, lasting for at least one month. Individually they can be devastating, and collectively they are very potent if untreated.

- **Intrusive recollections, such as:**
    - Nightmares
    - Flashbacks
    - Feeling the traumatic event is recurring
    - Intense psychological or physiological reactions when reminded of the event

- **Avoidance/numbing reactions, such as:**

  - Avoiding emotions, locations, or people associated with the trauma, including partner, hospitals, and caregivers
  - Avoiding situations in which it can recur
  - The brain choosing to forget the event, mimicking amnesia of parts of the event
  - Diminished interest in significant activities
  - Displaying detachment from others
  - Inability to feel loving feelings; sense of foreshortened future

- **Hyper-arousal, for instance:**

  - Having difficulty with sleep
  - Irritability or angry outbursts
  - Difficulty concentrating
  - Hyper-vigilance; exaggerated startle response; panic attacks or symptoms

- **Functional impairment, such as:**

  - Disassociation, which can often be display as lack of interest in any activity, including caring for the baby
  - Can present as significant distress in social, occupational, or other areas of functioning

The effect of these signs and symptoms can be debilitating and burdensome to affected mothers and it can affect their families. A significant number of women who have had a traumatic birth do not develop PTSD; why some are more prone to it is relatively unknown. However, studies report rates of PTSD after childbirth as varying between 1.5 and 9 percent of all births (*Breslau, N.* et al.; 2004). The differences among the research and its findings partly explained by differences in study designs, assessment tools, study populations according to Stramrood, C.et al; (2010), and usual maternity care practices and caregiver attitudes towards the mothers, babies or both cited by H. Goer (2010).

Those who have traumatic births but are not diagnosed with PTSD have fewer symptoms of the disorder, or the duration of symptoms was less than a month. These women are referred to variously as having post-traumatic stress symptoms (PTSS), post-traumatic stress effects (PTSE), or partial post-traumatic stress disorder (PPTSD) (N. Breslau et al., 2004). These terms refer to a less severe manifestation of birth trauma, meaning the mothers had some symptoms of PTSD, but not enough to qualify for a diagnosis. It is always wise to seek professional help when in doubt. Nursing these signs and symptoms in isolation is not advisable, but consider booking in for birth debriefing shortly after birth. The notion of women neglecting their needs and choosing to care for their families first, during other times is understandable and could be perceived as the standard. However, pregnancy, delivery, and post-natal periods can be demanding, and as such putting your needs and well-being first is, equally important. It is paramount for the care of the family, especially the new arrival in the household. Seek the appropriate support and graciously accept it from people that offers it. Bear in mind that recovery from these illnesses occurs with time and support, and can be facilitated by empathic discussion with a knowledgeable caregiver and various non-pharmacological treatments, such as:

- Relaxing bodywork/massage
- Adequate sleep
- Stretching exercise
- Secular yoga (neither religious nor spiritual practise form), with deep, but controlled breathing
- Support groups, Psychotherapy, counselling, and social work *(Skibniewski-Woods, 2011; Gamble, J. et al., 2005)*
- Help guides to trauma recovery. In the age of opulent digital information, one can explore self-help guides in the form of books, blogs, and social media.

Enjoy Life as a New Parent

Many parents want the answers to a stress-free and balanced life. The irony is that stress is part of life at varying degrees, and viewed as necessary or as a wake-up call. To figure out what one should or should not do can be daunting and challenging. A better insight into what will make one's life easier, that is, completely free of stress and the role of the mother much more enjoyable is ongoing. Some debates on stress explored socially and clinically, to gain a better insight into its management. Admitting one's limitation would not necessarily put the person under the spotlight, and it is okay to take things easy, but ensure that you have plans on which to fall back – for example, a network of friends and family to assist you. It is a matter of gaining perspective and loving how an individual has become through the process, as a new parent.

Eliminate Stress

Mothers often try to do their best in such a manner that compromises their health, which can result in all sorts of illness. It does not matter who the individual is, how old their kids are, or what your lifestyle is – sometimes parenting is just hard. It can be full of stress, but the truth is that it does not have to be so. No mother wants to look and feel stressed in the manner portray by the following image. However, envisage to actively managing stressful situations in such a manner that is less disruptive, engaging and at the same time, motivational. Manage this state of mind as quickly as possible and as effective, to avoid further health implications that could affect other family members.

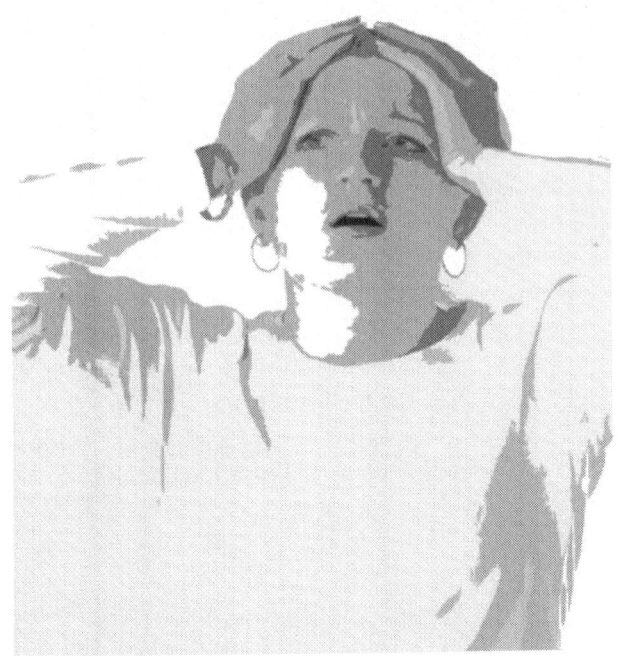

Outlook of a Stressful Mother

Balancing It All and Having Trouble Doing So

It can be troubling to balance everything, and doing the very best in a given day can make one feel like floating in place. It is a common sentiment shared amongst parents everywhere and yet so few discuss it. Consequently, the art of parenting is unique in all circumstances; it is an entirely new dynamic and trying to balance it all can be very challenging. Do not feel like a failure because; you are not alone, endeavour to resolve the challenge without the need to subscribe to medication.

Set Realistic Expectations

Choosing to reduce one's workload can influence positively on stress level and its associated illnesses. Things become harder to juggle when we take on more than we can handle. When a person takes on undue tasks in their professional lives, it is to advance, in the hope to provide a better life for our families. However, though women are multi-taskers, the toll on one's personal lives can be insurmountable, especially during the period immediately after birth. Pertinent to this is one role that matters and that will be what a legacy is all about as a parent. It is achievable with the right guidance, although, individuals may believe that, this is easier said than done. Cutting back on personal workload is highly advisable and do not be sentimental about doing so.

It is acceptable to drop all juggling balls and relax or take a break, until such a moment that the new mother is ready and prepared to continue. Some women probably realize that they have not taken a step back to gain perspective in this way. They go about their days with their heads down, doing whatever work they have. It is time to take a step back, take a deep breath, and see if these feelings or thoughts sound familiar:

- The feeling of the sense of work stacking up and never ending, or feeling as though one is missing-out on some major aspect of their baby's life is not uncommon. The intention to do the best that an individual can are noble, with all of the different roles, could make a person feel like failing at something. It is more than likely that the person is doing just fine, but the stress of it all can be overwhelming.

- The perception as impossible of balancing everything can be very difficult at times. Struggling through the list of tasks can be frustrating when the thought of catching-ups feels next to impossible. Do not feel like a failure at tasking and, therefore, balance is not part of your vocabulary. It gets better, and it helps to know that some women struggle with the same idea of balancing in order to achieve a healthy and happy lifestyle.

- There will be another day to get the task done, so when the body demands rest, take it as soon as possible. There can never be enough hours in the day to get everything done. A typical example, metaphorically, is even as a superwoman burning the midnight oil, it could impinge on one's ability to function well, and more often with the danger of compromising your own health. If the latter happens, who will care for your baby?

Working all hours, late into the night may results in everyone suffering, so it never feels like it is enough. It is frustrating when the basic chores are left undone, with so many women insisting on the perfect lifestyle, just like the one they had before given birth. Everything changes, hope is for the better, remember to keep the wits, and not lose it. The stress, the anxiety, and even the depression can weigh heavily on a woman who is trying so hard, only to feel that nothing achieved through one's efforts. It is frustrating, but there are effective ways in this book to make the most of a person's roles and finally feel like a true success in their life. Consequently, learn how to manage stress and take control of your life, which is paramount to your well-being.

Do ascribe to making a list, with a view to working in an organized fashion. Consider letting go of some tasks for a short while. It is common knowledge that prioritizing is an effective approach to multi-tasking. It is highly recommended and relevant in this instant, in the quest for a happy household and balance stress free life. Wherefore, women must, recognize that they can only do their best, and sometimes putting less pressure on themselves is the perfect way forward.

It is also practical to keep a diary of the features in an individual's daily life that one has a difficult time balancing. One of the options is to create various questions to analyse the areas that need more input; that is, professional ones. Do let go of little things. What are they?

Do plan to make your day work better for you, and avoid reaching a breaking point. In the light of the stress and challenges, in trying to balance it all, effectively, it is wise to seek help as soon as possible. It is okay to struggle initially to grasp the practical aspects of parenthood, even when the person has memorized the theoretical aspects very well. Permit me to assure you that, perfecting the theory of parenting is a lifetime process, so by no means feel like a failure, especially by someone else's standard. Indeed, there are right ways to achieve one's own perfection, and maintaining the standard that you personally set is achievement in its own right. Keep with it and do not give up. It is necessary now to feel good personally, having implemented the tips on managing stress, and it is okay recognising that you are doing your best.

- The idea of having it all as a necessity and not a nicety is the reality of the few; this is far from the grasp of most in the society. Some want to have it all, and now it is an actual expectation and demand from society. Do not permit others who may engage one in unprofitable affairs to expect you to be perfect. If a person set high expectations hoping for miracles and fail to live up to them, the guilt of the struggle to balance all of the various areas of one's overscheduled life can inevitably crush your own dreams.

Stress can lead to untold anxiety, which leads to frustration and often depression – and this is not a good equation to be in while nursing a baby. The truth is that many times these frustrations seem quite overwhelming, but rest assured, you are not alone. It is encouraging to rise above the challenges and take matters in its stride.

Learn to Manage It All

Those who have been through adversity or even tragedy will attest that, it is all about taking back one's life. It is no different; do learn to manage stress before it manages you. It may not sound easy; however, these tips are steps to staying focused on the end goal.

- Learn to truly prioritize, bearing in mind that, there is always room for improvement.
- Manage the stress – never give in to it. The way that one internalize the stress that is felt is up to the person. Any deal in life has the potential to be stressful, but it is all about how they are managed in our lives. Do not allow the daily stress to overwhelm at any point in time.

It is necessary to make a choice to learn how to manage the stress, prioritize, and stay ahead of it rather than giving in to it. The person at this point is in much better position to deal with the daily activities, of caring for their family. This is an important realization that can better equip one as a new mother. It is by changing the way that an individual manages things, a person's life in the process is ultimately changed, for better or worse.

- Listening to one's dedicated partner for support, and acknowledge the plight to influence it positively. Be subtle but approach the issue more directly; it will work out to your advantage.

- Take the time to get to know your partner by dedicating time for yourself to his life in a way that will work best for both of you. Then you can figure out how to achieve that balance and how to manage your stress level without recourse to medication.

- Endeavour to manage time as efficiently as possible to reduce stress levels. It does not mean staying up until all hours to get everything done, but the person does learn to make use of their time efficiently. Do consider delegation of duties whenever applicable and appropriate, leaving the person to take on other things in the household.

- Manage time as efficiently and responsibly, keep a detailed schedule and envisage what you can truly do through the day. Be honest and practical (listening to one's body is crucial), take a break when tired, and try to organise your day efficiently to make it all work.

- Changing one's outlook, attitude, and positive view of the world and everything in it is inspirational to the onlookers. Do not feel overwhelmed and stressed whenever there is a challenge in your life. Learn to approach it with an analytical mind (e.g., why, who, how, where, when) and explore what is next. Bear in mind that not all challenges have a negative impact. Some will pay off handsomely, whilst, others would not. However, deal with the problem directly and in the best possible way; this includes calling in the support network of families, friends, or caregivers. If feeling overwhelmed at every little thing, the level of anxiety will intensify, thereby; compound the situation. An individual must find a way to remain positive and to calm down; some duties and even daily chores can wait. Remember, there are other people in your situation, so you are not alone.

The stress of work in one's life balance can suck one in sometimes. In addition, it can cause an individual to feel like a bad parent or worker. It can take away one's productivity and cause a person to feel almost numb from the overwhelming feeling of trying to keep it all together. Remember, children love their parents and need them, and so prioritization becomes one of the keys to success as a good parent. It does not mean that work does not matter, but rather that; mothers should learn how to take control and manage stress rather than let it manage them. It also means that, mothers should take control over their lives and learn how to apply the prioritization tips to make it work.

Get Rid of Stress

The following infographics illustrates some stress impediments, management and steps to achieving a less stressful state of wellbeing. This state might be associated with both mild and severe forms of stress. Wherefore, the underlined texts represent combination of further impediment and blissful state of mind. If unmanaged, it could progress into other aspects of illnesses and loss of financial or social status.

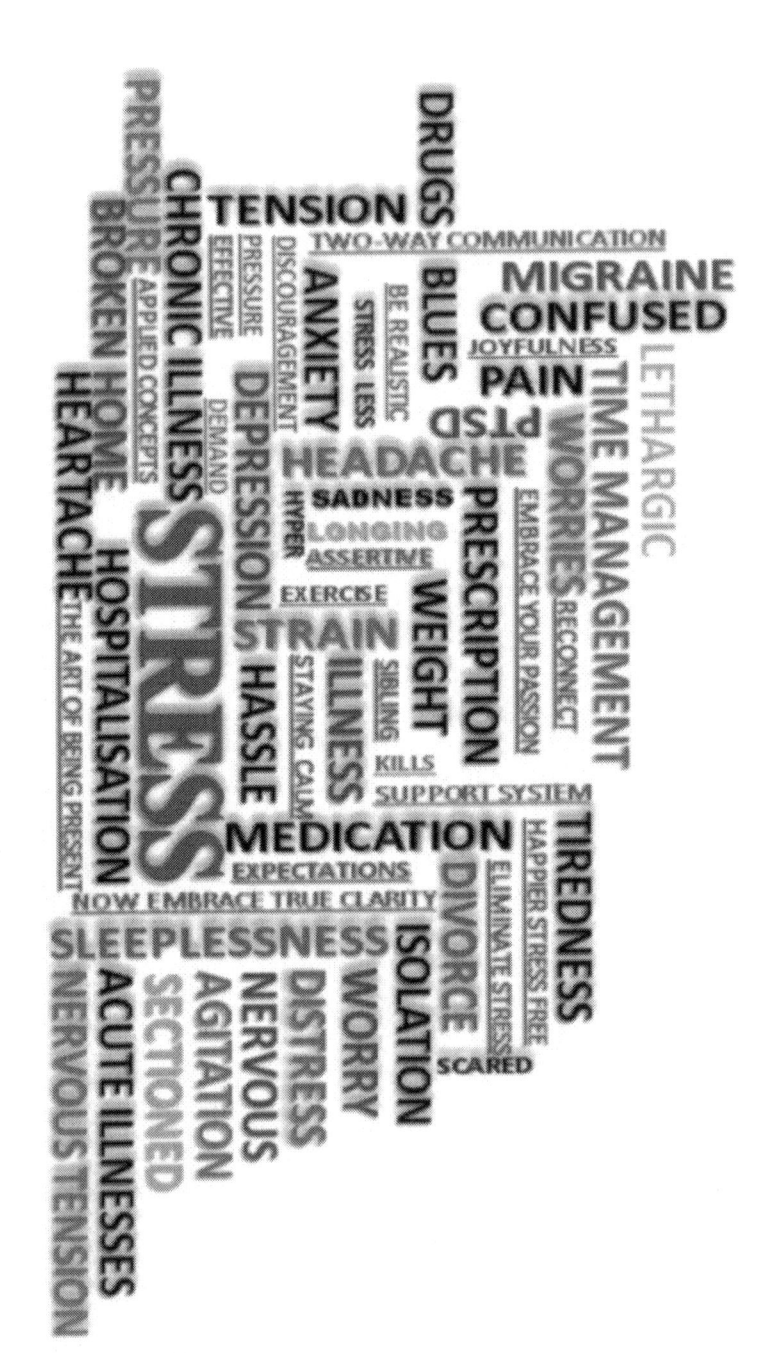

Every individual experience, adversities, triumphs, and defeats at some point in their lives; although some may seem obvious, they may take a while to fine tune. That is, to be better prepared for any adversity or defeat in the future. It is inspirational to have the desire to want to change and manage stress; this is the first and most important step in the journey. Consequently, knowing that one wants to change and that the person wants to make the stress outdated, this is, what matters. These elements are what makes life and the person's role of parenting that one dreamt happening.

1. The Art of Being Present

Quite simply put, this means that wherever a person is, *be there*, hopefully, this makes sense. Be present in the moment, and in body, spirit, soul, and mind. Share some much-needed quality time with your partner; this applies to being there physically or emotionally, to appreciate what you currently have.

Appreciate moments as its being experienced, keep reminding yourself of that, as the person go through the day. When an individual takes the time to be present, it means that they are truly engaged, with the moment that they are there and committed to what is happening as they experience it. It may sound easy enough, thinking the person is truly present, but take a step back, and they may realize that they are not present in most of the things that they do throughout the day. Could it be that, the person is floating all day long?

The other matter with being present is the aspect of not multitasking all day long and always worrying about what is next. It is okay to put other duties aside, even just for a moment, in order to be 'at the moment' for one's family. They do feel isolated and may feel that the new baby is getting all the attention, which is true, and it is because babies depend on parents in their helpless state. A word of warning; a person may choose to believe or not, that jealousy in varying degrees exists in their partner relating to the baby.

There may be the occasional exception, when being present for one's partner may be overruled by the need of the baby. It is okay, and hopefully they will understand and make the necessary adjustments. It is a hard adjustment at first, but when a person put the rest of the world on hold for that moment, and then get to experience life as it happens, it is wholesome; not just float through it. It is truly achievable and is worthwhile for a person's wellbeing and aspirational lifestyle.

2. Staying Calm

This indeed, could be easier said than done, staying calm when the baby is crying. The fact remains that the person need to cultivate staying in control for them and the baby's sake. The baby can sense stress from the mother; consequently, walking around in a cloud all day attracts both physical and mental confusion. It can affect one's family, especially, the baby in this crucial developmental stage. The price of physical and mental confusion may never be quantifiable or connected to this period of its life, when it is most vulnerable. Think hard about it; the more stress a person maintains on a daily basis, the more that is going to filter into their everyday life. It certainly carries over one's parenting style as you work to maintain a balance that never manifest.

It may be next to impossible for some women to stay calm in certain circumstances or environments that are too busy. They could perceive staying calm as impractical and elusive. The thought that everything has to be done right now and done perfectly every time by a new mother can result in illness beyond anxiety and prolonged depression. There is probably no such thing as saving something for later, and consequently the situation could transform into something that is chaotic, stressful, and anything but calm.

Delegating at this point is highly recommended for self-preservation and maintaining balance in your household and your life. Taking control of your life ought not to be perceived as a control freak, or a feeling of a sense of guilt over trying to be both a perfect mother and lover to your partner. It is a very common problem in the lives of some women, and it could be the main reason they walk around stressed all the time. Delegate, postpone, or plan a workable alternative. Admittedly, learning to stay calm may require some significant time in order to adjust to the new baby, but it gets better.

It is essential to stay calm even in very stressful situations or other life circumstances, remaining calm can work in your favour. *(Johnston, R.I et al 2004)*

Staying calm is something important to remember not only as a parent, but also in life. It is very easy being caught up in some form of stress, and the constant stream of too stressful activities in a person's life can inhibit their ability to be successful. To create a foundation for an all-around good, balanced life, learn to remain calm. *(Creedy, D.K et al; 2002)*

3. Find and Embrace True Clarity

In order to find and achieve clarity of mind by seeking out what is important, the person need to listen to a long and trusted inner voice, and this is okay. However, the list of the person's immediate priority will probably need further evaluating to reduce it a bit further. Taking off some tasks of what one perceives as truly important to achieve clarity is acceptable. Perhaps, when an individual personally defines clarity to fit the plan, they should focus on prioritization of the areas that requires immediate attention. In a sense, imagine it in such a manner sorted best to the individual.

The stress gradually melts away when one have both calmness and clarity, which often complement each other. It is acceptable to maintain both to feel good about accomplishing tasks, either personally or professionally, and applying the same principle.

A person may be stretched shortly after birth, may equally feel too busy and have no time to think about clarity. Though it may mean different things to different people, the point is, it is a necessary part of eliminating stress from one's role as a new mother. Do not be alarmed, by the fact that, you may need to take things more easily for a short while; listen to your body to maintain balance in life.

By getting in touch with that clarity, a person is focused, able to remain calm, and constantly gaining an important perspective on the pattern of the baby's needs. The person is adopting a suitable regime to perform even daily tasks. It is necessary to prioritise and learn how to manage life in order to allocate time for some enjoyment and happiness.

4. Find and Use Your Support System

One cannot emphasize enough the importance of a support system. To engage this tool, take advantage and be assertive, whether delegating or seeking help from a caregiver. In view of this, not wanting to ask for help, or feeling inadequate at this point, could be a terrible mistake. It could be that the person feels too proud to ask for help and very sure that you can handle it all. Maybe envisaged that they will be perfectly fine. It could also translate to feeling vulnerable and presenting this outlook as a sign of weakness. To be candid, life would be easier if one venture out of their comfort zone and ask for a little help now and again. Although, everyone in this time of transition should seek help, many people do not access the available support networks. It could be detrimental to their health and wellbeing.

It is necessary to enrol as many people in the support system as possible, in order to offset the burden of daily tasks, and thereby relieve stress. Simply having somebody come over to help with a simple task or to care for other children (if applicable); while the person tackles another job can be a lifesaver. There is nothing wrong with leaning on a support system – in fact, it is highly recommended. If the right people were to enlist in the support system, then it makes the individual's day much easier and more enjoyable.

Do not underestimate the spirit of humanity. Imagine how truly powerful it would be to have the right people to rely on now and again. To advocate trusting everyone enough to be part of the support system is not recommended; it does need to be the right people to make it work. It is important to envisage when it makes sense to seek their help and pertinent to discuss these issues with one's partner. They might have another insight into identifying the friends and family members that are close enough to assist, when the need may arise.

Whatever the task, a good support system is what you can lean on when you need that extra lift. The prospect of having a support system in place can help the individual to feel much better; it can take away a major source of stress in the end, as well. Asking for help is not an admission of failure, but rather a very wise move as a new mother. The reality is that no one can do it all, and sometimes an individual will need a little help. By finding the right people to create a support system, ensures that a person does so and feel good about it. Be careful selecting people for a support system and know that leaning on them sometimes a necessity and highly recommended part of parenting.

5. Effective, Assertive, and Two-Way Communication

The invaluable task of maintaining or building a two-way conversation with one's partner could be daunting and should not be underestimated. It is a skill for all parents to aspire to have in order to reduce the strain of communication. Consequently, assertive communication together with active listening can help to build confidence in varying degrees. Having established an effective two-way communication, be very assertive at all times when necessary using this tool, then create a long-lasting and close relationship in your life.

One of the greatest sources of parenting stress is anticipating the person that their child grows up to be. The fear of the unknown could aggravate stress and compound the status of the mind. No matter how busy or stressful life gets, having the ability to communicate with each other, verbally or otherwise, surpasses any hired aid. To this reason one places, a major emphasis, so learn how to communicate well with your partner, and eventually with the baby. It is paramount that an open line of communication be maintained, which is pivotal to staying connected; it is how a person could keep close to their partner and always stay an active part of their life.

6. Happier and Stress Free

The idea of first taking care of oneself is pertinent as far as self-preservations is concerned. What does it mean to be self-preserved and yet selfless? The characteristics or urge to protect oneself from difficulties or danger is self-preservation, according to the *Cambridge*

Dictionary. However, the content to which this word applies in this instance does not suggest abandoning one's role as a mother entirely and indulging in unprofitable affairs of selfishness. Moreover, it means that when a person is healthy, stress-free, and happy, then they can better take care of others. It is perhaps obvious and yet, probably overlooked by many, for one reason or the other. Trying these tips will eventually ensure that the person will be much happier and healthier, and you will leave a well-balanced life with less stress. It is wise to put aside an hour or so to dedicate to yourself; use it to catch up on some reading or to relax. Invest wisely in this time. This time could be to meet up with a friend or two or simply for a workout. Whatever activity you choose to indulge in, do not procrastinate, – just do it. Even having just a few moments to breathe and see the world from a different vantage point can be exhilarating. It is not a plan to take valuable time away from the baby – in fact, you can take the baby with you if venturing out. It is simply rewarding yourself for an accomplishment or finding a way to do something that you enjoy. In addition, it is highly recommended for an individual's mental health and your ability to cope.

The idea that women are perceived as caretakers by nature (denoting that taking care of everyone around them) but often neglect to take time to care for themselves is the norm. Reality dictates that a quick burnout is inevitable, and eventually stress and depression can occur as well.

It is important to indulge a little sometimes and to occasionally, put some time aside to do something that is personally good, as an individual. It may sound counterintuitive when everyone in the household relies on the individual for one thing or the other, but the bottom line is that time dedicated to taking care of yourself, as a person is relative and pays dividends. It ultimately makes one happier, healthier and much better mother in the process.

7. Embrace Your Passion

It is inevitable that the baby requires much attention in childhood, hope this aspect is accounted for during the process of planning of pregnancy, and birthing of the baby, irrespective of support networks and hired aids. If it turns out to be a personal passion, then stick to it and carve out a niche within to further build upon it. Consequently, it simply advocates occupying one's time with a certain passion. Keep busy to keep the devil at bay, so do not remain idle.

The reality is that mothers should find something that they are passionate about, use their imaginations to think up ideas, and stir up their innate intuition. It is of course before returning to work, assuming the individual has a job to which you are returning. It is well known that, women are intuitive (one of the greatest talents women possesses), imbued with many more ideas than their male counterparts are, and putting those ideas into practise is highly recommended.

It is lovely and great being a new mother and to have a purpose outside of this role is common. In addition, it is wise to get in touch with life's purpose and find what you feel passionate about; then you can fulfil this quest in your life. It could include a creative outlet by which the individual can enjoy some time to invest in their life. You may even uncover an ability to earn income outside of the norm, which makes the individual feel happy and fulfilled. Whatever personal steps taken have, the courage to seek advice, for both personal and professional inputs when necessary.

When a person explores a passionate idea and turns it into a professional or a lucrative hobby, it no longer feels like work. Find a happy, fulfilling, and content passion, where the individual can remain very excited and optimistic about what the future holds. Do not be discouraged, if confronted by obstacles; simply try again until you achieved your desired goals. However, do remain calm and access the support system without feeling as though the person have stretched herself too thin. The person can eventually, uncover some amazing potential and opportunities for immediate or future use.

8. Time Management

The use of time at every point in our lives at varying degrees is inevitable. However, managing time well can be a daunting task at times, but at best cost effective, nonetheless. The effect of poorly managed time will result in an inferior outcome even affecting health and overall wellbeing. A necessary component of being successful is the ability to manage one's time well. However, very often many forget or neglect to manage it. The effect of these build-ups, of mistakes can have devastating outcomes. It is plausible to lose one's ability to stay organised when; the person is metaphorically, pulled in different directions. However, not all is lost, and it is not too late to organise our tasks.

It is advantageous to plan and manage time in order to ensure a better outcome and increase your productivity. It may sound crazy to allot time to a person's tasks as well as delegate when needed, and to enjoy some time with your partner each day. Duly granted, managing personal time can undoubtedly take some effort, but it is a wise investment. It is sound to envisage the fact that time management can make one more efficient, effective, focused, and able to handle your daily tasks without feeling stress, exhaustion, and the terrible feeling of being overwhelmed. The truth is that the person at the process is learning to prioritize and manage their time more efficiently.

Time management translates to keeping a special list, as well as a calendar, which may help the person to remain focused and organised. What an individual may not realize is that time management is a vital part of parenting and life. It is essentially, at its best, organisational tool to possess. Although it may be different for everyone, the application of time management as an organisational tool is a critical part of being successful in this digital era and in keeping up with current affairs and trends. Time management does require some input at first, but it is reassuring that it becomes a seamless way of getting work done efficiently.

9. Reconnect with Sibling at Their Level

There is undeniable attention given to the new arrival in the household from family, friends, or caregivers. It can easily translate to varying degrees of jealousy from within and without the household. The level of trust needs evaluation, as such, due diligence against everyone the baby is being exposed to is highly recommended, even the immediate family.

Family members, especially siblings, observe how the baby is taking attention away from them, and this can translate as a direct threat to them; as such, they could proceed to resent the baby. Establish a two-way communication, encouraged by inspirational insight of siblings, in order to deal with this matter or similar ones. There is no right or wrong approach to this matter; it is best to keep them well informed. In the meantime, proactively safeguard the baby at all times, albeit in a subtle way, to reflect its helpless state and its dependency on adults.

Whether or not the new mother shares a close relationship with the baby's siblings, children can be unpredictable, so reaffirm that you love them as much as their sibling baby. It may ease the transition and worth a try. The nurture and nature of the siblings will determine their future outcome, and parenting is a lifetime learning curve. Take it in its stride and develop a connection that will foster a healthy relationship with the siblings. Remember to tap into the support system discussed earlier. The siblings' perception of this transitional period and the sense of feeling threaten may well be overrated, but should not be underestimated. Consequently, even when the mother is feeling progressive, the truth is that there is usually a rather large gap in generational thinking and views of the world. Acknowledging the existence of this gap and working towards finding a common ground will make the transition period endurable.

10. Application of These Concepts

The previous chapter 'Me Time' explore certain concept relating to how mothers could deal with stress following pregnancy and birth. However, it is an opportunity to put into motion these tips and constantly evaluate practical options that does not increase stress, but lessens it. It is possible to eliminate some of the stress of parenting in life. The advocacy of using a support system is a good concept, and understanding the balance is something that an individual must work towards and try to achieve. This idea all makes sense in theory, so work on putting them into practice. It requires adjustments and work, but they are necessary investments and worthwhile.

The time to put these concepts into current dynamics and make some changes could not come sooner, especially if things have not previously worked out. There is no promise that it will be easy, but it is certainly worthwhile to try. It will certainly make the person, their partner and children happier, creating a less stressful and enjoyable life.

Adopt these theories and put them into practice through the following ideas and guidelines.

- Although from a professional point of view and inspired personal experience, it helps to think through how these concepts can truly work in one's life. Admittedly, mothers can identify with at least one of the concepts presented in the guidelines, adopting them to reflect their personal situation in any given moment is prudent. It is ultimately being very honest with yourself to achieve the clarity needed for this journey of discovery, though it could be difficult at the beginning, but nevertheless worth it.
- Consider the adjustments that it needs, and prioritize or scale back in certain areas of activities. There is a certain degree of commitment and dedication required to make many a sacrifice of this nature to work in one's life. A crucial adjustment will lead to a better outcome for all parties involved.
- Let us acknowledge that taking stress out of the equation takes time and commitment from the onset. These changes are not going to happen overnight, so one must be patient and dedicated. The changes will occur as much as an individual place their energy on it (denoting every effort placed in making it happen), with visible aspects taking hold when one take the time to adjust and live with it. Whilst some changes may mean instant gratification, others may take a little time to manifest.

The time has come for the person to get rid of the negative or potentially toxic elements of one's current life. Aspire to seize a positive outlook at every opportunity and keep calm, be inspired and endeavour to inspire people. If a person is unhappy with having little time for themselves, then they need to make time. If an individual feels frustrated due to negative influences, then it is time to get rid of them in a pragmatic manner. It might sound easier said than done, but it is necessary to one's long-term success, and this is one way to feel happier about your outlook and your life moving forward. Getting rid of negativity allows the positive energy to dwell into a person's life.

The motivation to create a lifestyle that grants happiness surrounds a person in one's environment, access it, and tap into it to gain insight into your aspirations. Stress should not be anyone's regular state of mind, and to eliminate it requires diligent work. If an individual is constantly feeling anxious, depressed, stressed, or resentful, it is not a lifestyle for parenting. The wellbeing of that person is essentially compromised, lowering their immune system, thereby, exposing them to all kinds of both chronic and acute illnesses. If some dynamics (equilibrium of body) is off, choose to change in order to achieve long-lasting happiness. The role of parenting ought not to be stressful. It is then logical to create a lifestyle that personally works well, and accommodates beyond reasoning, the individuals whom you love.

Furthermore, recognize what is not working and then be ready to make the necessary adjustments. The moment has come for you to take the plunge and step up for a great ride towards your ultimate dream of a less stressful life; this should include banishing anxiety, which should not knock at your door after this process. There is no such thing as easy and free attainment in life that is valuable to groups or individual, so if a person want the prize, keep your eye on it. Parenting without anxiety is amazing, though a little stress now and again can build up one's character; this may seem counterintuitive, but truly, it is not.

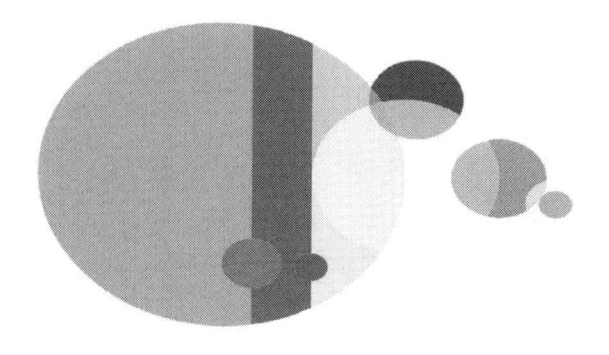

SUMMARY

Congratulations on completing one or all of the task and for persevering with the steps taken to earn this achievement, specifically, the newborn baby rubdown. There is a learning curve, but it is an experience worth cherishing in motherhood and beyond. It is with hope that by passing on an experience to the next generations and sharing it amongst friends and families, a beacon of history and tradition can meet modern practises, especially, in this context.

The growing source of information in digital media and increasingly the sophistication of newer versions of such media can be daunting. However, searching for any word or research material in a search engine will produce many results. The advent of social media denotes the full or partial digital exploration of business or pleasure. The mode has exponentially propelled digital sharing of information in modern times, with the World Wide Web (www) at its helm. The personal use of these media to gain information on many topics is unavoidable, including health related, amongst others and general news broadcast. In addition, using this mode to gain information is universally acceptable and well documented. In some remote parts of the world, the access of medical information through remote digital aid are growing in popularity and fiercely advocated by healthcare professionals. The source enhances the knowledge needed by the caregiver. It ensures that they are less isolated from current medical breakthroughs and mothers are better informed of their care plan. Mothers are cautiously encouraged to explore the digital media for information that can improve the overall quality of life for them and their families.

The principle of practising is to perfect one's experience in their endeavour; do practise until confident enough to fulfil the task. The views of clinicians on the importance of the unique newborn rubdown and subsequent bath, in relation to its acclaimed prevention of malodorousness beyond childhood, though mixed but nonetheless encouraging. It is with great hope that a further exploration of the scientific base of this claim is disseminated in subsequent editions, in order to gain a better insight into the composition of the property responsible for eliminating body odour. Medically, it has been neither clinically substantiated nor disproved. An instigation of a robust research to prove or disprove the acclaimed benefits, especially the properties of palm oil action against bacteria that causes malodorousness is pending. The findings will be available in subsequent editions.

A personal certainty in the benefits of the newborn rubdown is the result of one's experience and attested by many. However, no research currently disapproved its safety or benefits. The palm oil derivatives give its credibility in its various purpose, especially, in cleansing, when use in accordance with the unique newborn baby massage and subsequent bath to mention but a few. The question at this moment is whether it warrants trying this unique baby rubdown for one or more of its benefits. Whatever the decision, hope it is inspirational, as the goal is to promote health and wellbeing through this technique, together with practical tips to reduce stress and better manage one's time, mentioned in previous chapters.

It is hoped that by re-enforcing the overall awareness of the use of abdominal massage in older babies has inspired many mothers. Clinicians worldwide endorsed the technique to relief colic, and mothers who have experienced it fiercely attest to its benefits. The tips on managing personal time well, to improve the quality of life and to minimise the stress of parenting are all from numerous source, including, personal life experience. It is also prudent to explore the topics in more details with your professional caregivers at any stage. These tips are intended as the first option and the exploration of other drastic measures, such as drugs, as a last resort (after considerable consultation with a medical practitioner such as, your general practitioner).

General Critique

The West resisted the Eastern practises of acupuncture until recently and universally, still divided on the benefits and clinical relevance to its claims. These doubts are based neither on robust studies nor on adversity coursed by the method itself. The efficacy of any procedure must not, be based only on known clinical or pharmaceutical impact, but it should also be given the benefit of the doubt until proven otherwise. The critique of this book is relevant and inevitable with anticipated, controversial comments of the likelihood of media bashing, with respect to its content and claims. It is my hope that debates will open up around the issues raised within, especially, amongst mothers themselves.

The hypothesis which is based on the safety and the use of the procedure in many parts of the world, except perhaps in Western countries; the conducted study reinforces the true benefits of the method. The main benefit is measurable in adulthood, many years into the future. However, it is common for controversial issues to either be upheld or completely dismissed by both consumers and the media, in the light of the lack of previous research and the perceived benefits of the claim. Consequently, here is an open invitation to groups or individuals to provide constructive comment; to any issue raised within the subject of newborn rubdown and the special tips for mothers. Their opinions may resolve any doubt of the reliability of the perceived benefits and as such, essential to mothers. This critique is important and perhaps paramount; either way its endorsement is equally essential to reassure consumers.

In summary, whether one is a first-time mother or simply a mother again, take great pleasure in enjoying the moments with the baby. There is no greater duty or joyfulness than being a mother; a fact often ignored by some in our society. The challenges in life are learning curves, to even, pass onto the future generations, or just accept them as another experience for personal or professional attainment. Finally, it is with great pleasure and humility with view to; wish mothers all the best and most of all to enjoy stress-free parenthood.

NOTES

BIBLIOGRAPHY

1. Weerapong, Pornratshanee, Hume, Kolt (2005): "The Mechanisms of Massage and Effects on Performance, Muscle Recovery and Injury Prevention" Sports Medicine **35** (3): 235-256.
2. UNICEF UK (2013) "The evidence and rationale for the UNICEF UK Baby Friendly Initiative standards" 4 (4.2) pp 54.
3. WHO; The Definition of Newborn baby, source: World Health Organisation (2013) www.who.int.topics/infant_newborn/en.
4. Oxford Dictionary; The Definition of Newborn, source: Oxford Dictionaries.com (2013)
5. Definition of massage (Online-Boots WebMD) (2013) (www.medterms.com.)
6. Odent, M. (2002) First Hour following Birth. Don't Wake The Mother! Retrieved 2014 online www.midwiferytoday.com Issue 61.
7. What is Massage Therapy? (2013) Retrieved online- Altmedicine.about.com.
8. Online Etymology Dictionary, massage (etymonline.com).
9. Merriam Webster; Online Dictionary, massage Retrieved (2013) (m-w.com).
10. Calvert, R. (2002-04-01). World: Healing Arts Press
11. "Massage Therapy as CAM." The National Centre for Complementary and Alternative Medicine (NCCAM) 2006-09-01 Retrieved 2007-09-26.
12. "Policy for Therapeutic Massage in an Academic Health Centre: A Model for Standard Policy Development." The Journal of Alternative and Complementary Medicine 2007 Retrieved 2007-09-26. 13 (4) pp.471-475.
13. Beider S, Mahrer NE, Gold JI (December 2007). "Paediatric massage therapy: an overview for clinicians." Paediatric Clinical North Am. **54** (6): 1025–41; xii–xiii.
14. Hoath, Steven (2003). Neonatal skin: structure and function (2. ed., rev. and expanded. ed.). New York [u.a.]: Dekker. pp. 193-208. ISBN 0-8247-0887-3.

15. Wakai, RT; Lengle, JM; Leuthold, AC (2000 Jul). "Transmission of electric and magnetic foetal cardiac signals in a case of ectopia cordis: the dominant role of the vernix. caseosa." Physics in medicine and biology **45** (7): 1989-95. PMID 10943933.
16. Saunders C. The vernix caseosa and subnormal temperature in premature infants. Br J Obstetric Gynaecology 1948; 55:442–444.
17. Riesenfeld B, Stromberg B, Sedin G. The influence of vernix caseosa on water transport through semi permeable membranes and the skin of full-term infants. Neonatal Physiological Measurements: Proceedings of the Second International Conference on Foetal and Neonatal Physiological Measurements, 1984: 3–6.
18. Vickers A, Ohlsson A, Lacy JB, Horsley A (2004). "Massage for promoting growth and development of preterm and/or low birth-weight infants". Cochrane Database Syst Rev (2): CD000390.
19. Barr, RG (2002). "Changing our understanding of infant colic." Archives of paediatrics & adolescent medicine **156** (12): 1172–4. PMID 12444822.
20. Saavedra, Maria A.L.; Costa, Juvenal S. Dias da; Garcias, Gilberto; Horta, Bernardo L.; Tomasi; Mendonça, Rodrigo (2003). "Infantile colic incidence and associated risk factors: A cohort study." Jornal de Paediatrica **79** (2): 115–22. doi: 10.2223/JPED.962. PMID 14502331.
21. Lust, K. D.; Brown, J. E.; Thomas, W. (1996). "Maternal Intake of Cruciferous Vegetables and Other Foods and Colic Symptoms in Exclusively Breast-Fed Infants." Journal of the American Dietetic Association **96** (1): 46–48. doi: 10.1016/S0002-8223(96) 00013-2. PMID 8537569.
22. Wessel, MA; Cobb, JC; Jackson, EB; Harris Jr, GS; Detwiler, AC (1954). "Paroxysmal fussing in infancy, sometimes called colic." Paediatrics **14** (5): 421–35. PMID 13214956.
23. Barr, RG; Rotman, A; Yaremko, J; Leduc, D; Francoeur, TE (1992). "The crying of infants with colic: A controlled empirical description." Paediatrics **90** (1 Pt 1): 14–21. PMID 1614771.

24. Merriam-Webster online dictionaries Merriam-Webster Retrieved 2007-03-27. (Newborn).
25. Ekwenye, U.N and Ijeomah, Antimicrobial effects of palm kernel oil and palm oil King Mongkut's Institute of Technology Ladkrabang Science Journal, Vol. 5, No. 2, Jan-Jun (2005).
26. Reeves, James B.; Weihrauch, John L.; Consumer and Food Economics Institute (1979). Composition of foods: fats and oils. Agriculture handbook 8-4. Washington, D.C.: U.S. Dept. of Agriculture, Science and Education Administration. p. 4. OCLC 5301713.
27. Poku, Kwasi (2002). "Origin of oil palm". Small-Scale Palm Oil Processing in Africa. FAO Agricultural Services Bulletin 148. Food and Agriculture Organization. ISBN 92-5-104859-2.
28. Harold McGee. On Food And Cooking: The Science And Lore Of The Kitchen, Scribner, 2004 edition. ISBN 978-0-684-80001-1.
29. Cottrell, RC (1991). "Introduction: nutritional aspects of palm oil." The American journal of clinical nutrition **53** (4 Suppl): 989S–1009S. PMID 2012022.
30. US Federal Food, Drug & Cosmetic Act, 21 CFR 101.25 as amended in Federal Register July 19, 1990, Vol.55 No.139 pg.29472. (Retrieved 2013).
31. UK Food Labelling Regulations (SI 1984, No.1305) (Retrieved 2013-British Library).
32. Greenpalm.com. "What is Palm Oil?" 2010-06-05. Retrieved 2013-01-28.
33. "Palm Oil Continues to Dominate Global Consumption in" (2006/07) (Press release). United States Department of Agriculture. June 2006. Retrieved 22 September 2009.
34. Che Man, YB; Liu, J.L.; Jamilah, B.; Rahman, R. Abdul (1999). "Quality changes of RBD palm olein, soybean oil and their blends during deep-fat frying." Journal of Food Lipids **6** (3): 181–193. doi:10.1111/j.1745-4522.1999.tb00142.x.
35. Matthäus, Bertrand (2007). "Use of palm oil for frying in comparison with other high-stability oils." European Journal of Lipid Science and Technology **109** (4): 400. doi: 10.1002/ejlt.200600294.

36. Lian Pin Koh and David S. Wilcove (2007). "Cashing in palm oil for conservation." Nature **448**: 993–994.
37. Heller, Lorraine (16 December 2005). "Palm oil 'reasonable' replacement for trans fats, say experts." Food navigator. Retrieved 1 March 2013.
38. "Palm Oil Not A Healthy Substitute For Trans Fats, Study Finds." Science Daily Website: Science News. Science Daily LLC. 2009-05-11. Retrieved 2010-05-12.
39. Natasha Gilbert (4 July 2012). "Palm-oil boom raises conservation concerns: Industry urged towards sustainable farming practices as rising demand drives deforestation." Nature.
40. Morales, Alex (18 November 2010). "Malaysia Has Little Room for Expanding Palm-Oil Production, Minister Says." Bloomberg. Retrieved 1 March 2013.
41. Scott-Thomas, Caroline (17 September 2012). "French firms urged to back away from 'no palm oil' label claims." Food navigator. Retrieved 7 March 2013.
42. Kiple, Kenneth F.; Conee Ornelas, Kriemhild, eds. (2000). The Cambridge World History of Food. Cambridge University Press. ISBN 0521402166. Retrieved 30 August 2012.
43. Obahiagbon, F.I. (2012). "A Review: Aspects of the African Oil Palm (Elaeis guineesis Jacq.)." American Journal of Biochemistry and Molecular Biology: 1–14. doi: 10.3923/ajbmb.2012. Retrieved 30 August 2012.
44. British Colonial Policies and the oil palm industry in the Niger Delta region of Nigeria, 1900-1960.]." http://www.africa.kyotou.ac.jp/kiroku/asm_normal/abstracts/pdf/21-1/19-33.pdf African Study Monographs **21** (1): 19–33. 2000.
45. Bellis, Mary. "The History of Soaps and Detergents." "In 1864, Caleb Johnson founded a soap company called B.J. Johnson Soap Co., in Milwaukee. In 1898, this company introduced a soap made of palm and olive oils, called Palmolive." (www.about.com).
46. Hartley, C. W. S. (1988). The Oil Palm, 3rd edn. Longman Scientific and Technical, Harlow, U.K.

47. *Development of Palm Oil and Related Products in Malaysia and Indonesia Rajah Rasiah & Azmi Shahrin, University Malaya, 2006.*
48. *Sharing Innovating Experiences 5/Agriculture and Rural Development in the South, Chapter 1-Oil Palm R&D Malaysia United Nations Office For South-South Cooperation.*
49. *BBC Panorama. 22 February 2010. Retrieved 2010. "Palm oil products and the weekly shop".*
50. *Rosalie Marion Bliss (2009). "Palm Oil Not a Healthy Substitute for Trans Fats."*
51. *Edem, D.O. (2002). "Palm oil: Biochemical, physiological, nutritional, haematological and toxicological aspects: A review." Plant Foods for Human Nutrition (Formerly Qualitas Plantarum)* **57** *(3): 319–341. doi:10.1023/A:1021828132707.*
52. *"The truth about fats: bad and good." Health.harvard.edu. Retrieved 2013.*
53. *"Welcome to Tocotrienol Resource Website." Tocotrienol.org. Retrieved 2012.*
54. *Diet, Nutrition and the Prevention of Chronic Diseases, WHO Technical Report Series 916, Report of a Joint WHO/FAO Expert Consultation, World Health Organization, Geneva, (2003), p. 88 (Table 10).*
55. *Valuable minor constituents of commercial red palm olein: carotenoids, vitamin E, ubiquinones and sterols Bonnie Tay Yen Ping and Choo Yuen May, Journal of Oil Palm Research, Vol 12, No 1, June 2000, pg14-24*
56. *American Psychiatric Association (APA). (2000). Diagnostic and statistical manual of mental disorders (Revised 4th ed.). Washington, DC: APA.*
57. *Soet JE, Brack GA, DiIorio C. (2003). Prevalence and predictors of women's experience of psychological trauma during childbirth. Birth 30(1):36-46.*
58. *Breslau N, Lucia V, Davis G. (2004). Partial PTSD versus full PTSD: an empirical examination of associated impairment. Psychological Medicine 34(7): pp1205-1214.*
59. *Goer H. (2010). Cruelty in maternity wards: Fifty years later. Journal of Perinatal Education 19(3): 33-42.*

60. Johnston-Robledo I, Barnack J. 2004. Psychological issues in Childbirth. Women & Therapy 27(3-4):133-150.
61. Simkin P. 2011. Pain, suffering, and trauma in labour and prevention of subsequent posttraumatic stress disorder. Journal of Perinatal Education 20 (3): 166-176.
62. Stramrood C, Huis C, Van Pampus M, Leonard W, et al. 2010. Measuring posttraumatic stress following childbirth: a critical evaluation of instruments. Journal of Psychosomatics in Obstetrics and Gynaecology 31(1): 40-49.
63. Creedy DK, Horsfall J, Gamble J. (2002). Developing critical appraisal skills using a review of the evidence for postpartum debriefing. Aust J Midwifery 15(4):3-9.
64. Gamble JA, Creedy DK, Webster J, Moyle W. 2002. A review of the literature on debriefing or non-directive counselling to prevent postpartum emotional distress. Midwifery 8(1):72-9.
65. Gamble J, Creedy D, Moyle W, Webster J, McAllister M, Dickson P. 2005. Effectiveness of a counseling intervention after a traumatic childbirth: a randomized controlled trial. Birth. 32(1):11-19.
66. Skibniewski-Woods D. (2011). A review of postnatal debriefing of mothers following traumatic birth. Community Practice 84(12): 29-32.
67. Beck CT, Indman P. (2005). The many faces of postpartum depression. J Obstet Gynecol Neonatal Nurs 34(5):569-76
68. Cigoli V, Gilli G, Saita E. (2006). Relational factors in psychopathological responses to childbirth. J Psychosom Obstet Gynaecol 27(2):91-7.
69. Czarnocka J, Slade P. (2000). Br J Clin. Psychol. 39 (Pt 1):35-51.Prevalence and predictors of post-traumatic stress symptoms following childbirth.
70. Declercq E, Sakala C, Corry M, Applebaum S. (2008). New Mothers Speak Out: National Survey Results Highlight Women's Postpartum Experiences. Childbirth Connection: New York.
71. Gross MM, Hecker H, Keirse MJ. 2005. An evaluation of pain and "fitness" during labour and its acceptability to women. Birth 32(2):122-8.

72. Szalay S, (2011). *Post-Traumatic Stress Disorder after Childbirth in an Out-of-Hospital Birth Population*. Presentation at Annual Conference of Midwives Association of Washington State, Seattle, Washington (unpublished-retrieved online 2013).

73. Nicholls K, Ayers S. (2007). Childbirth-related post-traumatic stress disorder in couples: a qualitative study. Br J Health Psychol. 12(Pt 4):491-509.

74. Beck C. (2004). Post-traumatic stress disorder due to childbirth: the aftermath. Nursing Research 53(4): 216-24.

75. Elmir R, Schmied V, Wilkes L, Jackson D. 2010. Women's perceptions and experiences of a traumatic birth: a meta-ethnography. Journal of Advanced Nursing 66(10): 2142-53.

76. Rothschild B. (2010). *8 Keys to Safe Trauma Recovery: Take Charge Strategies for Reclaiming Your Life*. W.W. Norton & Co. Inc.: New York.

77. Cori JL. 2007. *Healing from Trauma: A Survivor's Guide to Understanding Your Symptoms and Reclaiming Your Life*. Marlowe & Company: Cambridge, MA.

78. Shapiro F. 2012. *Getting Past Your Past: Tale Control of Your Life with Self-Help Techniques from EMDR Therapy*. Rodale: New York.

79. Roberts DM, Ostapchuk M, O'Brien JG. Am Fam Physician. Infantile colic. (2004) Aug 15; 70(4):735-40. Review. PMID: 15338787.

80. Sung V., H. Hiscock, M. L. K. Tang, F. K. Mensah, M. L. Nation, C. Satzke, R. G. Heine, A. Stock, R. G. Barr, M. Wake. Treating infant colic with the probiotic Lactobacillus reuteri: double blind, placebo controlled randomised trial. BMJ, 2014; 348 (apr01 2): g2107 DOI: 10.1136/bmj.g2107.

81. The Dictionary of modern medicine. J.C. Segen's Medical 2012 Farlex, Inc

INDEX

A

Activity, *3*
admiration, *ix*
adolescent, *9, 103*
adulthood, *xiv, 16, 20, 99*
Africa, *9, 26, 32, 104*
antidote, *8*
APGAR, 3
Appearance, *3*
author, *xiv, 9, 20, 25, 31, 48, 58, 64, 99*

B

baby, ix, xiv, xvi, 1, 2, 3, 4, 5, 7, 8, 9, 12, 13, 15, 16, 17, 20, 21, 22, 25, 26, 27, 30, 31, 39, 40, 43, 45, 46, 48, 49, 50, 51, 52, 54, 55, 57, 58, 59, 60, 61, 72
Baby shower gel/wash, 50
Bask in the moment, 64
baths, *51, 52, 54, 55*
Bathtub time, 54
beacon of history, 97
benefits, *ix, xiii, xiv, 10, 13*, 15, 17, 20, *25, 26, 27, 34, 40, 42, 57, 61, 98*, 99
birth, *xv, 1, 2, 3, 4, 5, 9, 12, 19, 20, 25, 26, 30, 31, 60, 103*
blood circulation, 70
body odour, *xiv, 17*
burp, *21, 54*

C

Caesarean section, *3*
Camomile oil, 59, 62
cereals, 32

children, 12, 26, 61
clinically, 5, 9, 25
clinician, 27
clinicians, 16, 98
colic, *13, 20, 21, 22, 27, 103*
Colic, 21, 27, 103
commodity, 32, 35
complementary, *12*
controversial, *ix, 9, 15, 99*
conventional, *ix*
cosmetics, 32, 34, 40
Cotton wools, 40
counterintuitive, 76
crisps, 32
critique, 99
cultural fusion, *26*
culturally, *ix*, 25

D

dedicate, *ix, x*
development, *xv, 2, 16, 26, 42, 103*

E

efficacy, 34, 99
endearing, *ix*
endorsement, 99
ethically, *ix, 25*
ethically sourced, 32

F

foetuses, *2*
free radicals, 26
friction of kneading, *7*
fusion of cultural, 19

G

general practitioner, *3*
gimmick, *15*, *19*
gravitas, *19*
Greek, *7*
Grimace, *3*
groin, 45, 48
growth, *xv*, *26*, *42*, *103*

H

health and wellbeing, *xiii*, *xiv*
healthcare, *ix*, *xiii*, *xiv*, *xv*, *5*, *9*, *16*, *19*, *58*
heart, 71
hospital, *3*, *4*
humanity, *x*
hygiene, xiv, 19, 26, 40
hypothesis, 99

I

impossible, *x*
interesterification, 33
intestinal fluids, 71

J

journey home, *5*
joy, *xiii*, *xv*, *2*

L

labour, *xv*, *9*, *15*, *72*
Latin, *7*
lotions, 35, 40
lottery, *xv*
lymphatic, 70

M

malodorous, 35, 40
malodorousness, *xiv*, *25*, *98*
Malodorousness, 16, 25
manifest, *25*, *26*
margarine, 32
massage, xiii, xiv, 7, 8, 9, 12, 15, 16, 19, 20, 23, 25, 26, 27, 31, 39, 48, 49, 52, 57, 58, 59, 60, 61, 102
massage stokes, 71
mayonnaise, 34
Methodology, *16*
Methods, 29
midwife, xiii, xiv, xv, 2, 3, 23, 58
Mint oil, 59, 62
moaning, *ix*, *21*
motherhood, *97*
multiplication of bacteria, 26
Mum, 64
muscles, xi, 2, 7, 8, 70, 71

N

natural or non scented, 40
Newborn, viii, 1, 102, 104
NEWBORN BABY, viii
newborn baby massage, *57*, *60*
non-Wessel's, *22*

O

odour, *xiv*, *16*, *19*, *20*, *25*, *34*, *98*
olive oils, 35, 105
opportunities, *xv*
origin, *8*, *9*, *10*
Overseas, *xv*

P

paediatrician, *2*, *3*
Palm kernel oil, 39, 59, 62

111

palm oil, 12, 16, 32, 33, 34, 35, 40, 104, 105
Palm oil, 32, 34, 42, 105, 106
parents, *ix, xiii, xiv, xv, xvi, 1, 3, 8, 9, 10, 13, 15, 16, 17, 20, 23, 25, 26, 27, 61, 64, 72*
Partner, 64
pharmaceutical, 99
pharmacopeia, 21, 78, 82
pioneering, *15*
Post-Traumatic Stress Disorder, 74, 76, 108
Post-Traumatic Stress Effects,, 76
Post-Traumatic Stress Symptoms, 76
pragmatic, viii
    pragmatic, viii
pregnancy, 72
pregnant, *9*
professionals, *ix, xv, 2, 3, 20*
Pulse, *3*
purification, 33

Q

qualitative, *16*
Quantitative, *16*

R

randomised, *16*
reflex activity, *7*
relaxation, *7*
research, 5, 9, 13, 15, 27, 34, 98, 99
Respiration, *3*
rubdown, ix, xiii, 8, 9, 12, 15, 19, 25, 40, 98
RUBDOWN, *viii*

S

Safflower oil, 59, 62
Secular, 76

self-massage, 70, 71
shampoos, 35
slippery, 31
soap, 32, 40, 51, 52, 105
soaps, 32, 35, 42
society, *ix, 2, 3, 5, 9, 40*
special oil as lubricant, *20*
stronger, *ix, 64*
Sweden, *5*
sweets, 32

T

tearful, *2*
therapy, *8, 12, 102*
toiletries, 40
truck box, 60
tummy, 23, 45, 60

U

unequivocal, *xiii*

V

vernix, 26, 30, 31, 103
vernix caseosa, 26, 103
vibration, *8*

W

washing powders, 32
WHO, 35, 106
woman, *xiv*
worldwide, *x, 5, 99*
wound care, 34

Y

yoga, **76**

ABOUT THE AUTHOR

In the course of Bridget's career as a specialist healthcare professional, her roles in women's health were memorable and provided her with an added wealth of experience and extensive international exposure. Whilst she acquired aspects of project management later in her career, an enriched cultural intelligence (CQ) enhance the overall process in the strategic planning, developing, implementing, and evaluation of multinational projects.

Her pragmatic approach to delivering projects on time, to exacting specification, and her ability to negotiate complex tasks with leadership qualities is evident in her career. In addition, her experience in leadership and networking opportunities enhanced her overall professional prospect. She attained various research methodologies for professional applications, and the value of its use thereafter; including the dissemination of data was invaluable in the publication of Squeaky Clean.

Although, seen as an introvert, she is an intense observer and aspiring philanthropist. The author lives with her family and is a food critic. It is with great pleasure that she continues to explore relevant opportunities that will enhance the lives of people in the community, specifically, women empowerment. To this end, enjoy using the tips, along with the technique described, even the newborn baby rubdown. Indulge in the inspiration gain from within this context, no doubt unique to some and endeavour to use the tips on managing birth related stress.

Made in the USA
Charleston, SC
19 September 2015